# Special Ops
# Fitness Training

# Special Ops Fitness Training

**High-Intensity Workouts of Navy SEALs, Delta Force, Marine Force Recon and Army Rangers**

**MARK De LISLE**

photography by Andy Mogg

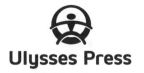

**Ulysses Press**

Published in the United States by Ulysses Press
P.O. Box 3440
Berkeley, CA 94703
www.ulyssespress.com

ISBN-13: 978-1-56975-582-2
Library of Congress Control Number 2006907935

Printed in Canada by Webcom

10 9 8 7 6 5

| Editorial/Production | Lily Chou, Claire Chun, Lauren Harrison, Judith Metzener, Steven Zah Schwartz |
| --- | --- |
| Index | Sayre Van Young |
| Cover design | what!design @ whatweb.com |
| Cover photographs | front: © iStockphoto.com |
|  | back: © Mark Divine and Tony Vernetti |
| Interior photographs | Andy Mogg, except on pages 3, 5, 6, 7, 8, 9, 10, 16, 18 © Mark Divine and Tony Vernetti |
| Models | Mark De Lisle, Mike De Lisle, Jeff Stephenson |

Distributed by Publishers Group West

Please Note
This book has been written and published strictly for informational purposes, and in no way should be used as a substitute for consultation with health care professionals. You should not consider educational material herein to be the practice of medicine or to replace consultation with a physician or other medical practitioner. The author and publisher are providing you with information in this work so that you can have the knowledge and can choose, at your own risk, to act on that knowledge. The author and publisher also urge all readers to be aware of their health status and to consult health care professionals before beginning any health program.

Thank you, Wendy and my family, for always being by my side; my heart will always be yours. Scott Joseph, thanks for having my back.

To all operators—active, retired, or having paid the ultimate sacrifice for this nation. You are an inspiration to me and this nation for your dedication, motivation, and desire to serve. Your families suffer greatly when you are away in training or combat. I hope all who serve in our military understand our gratitude.

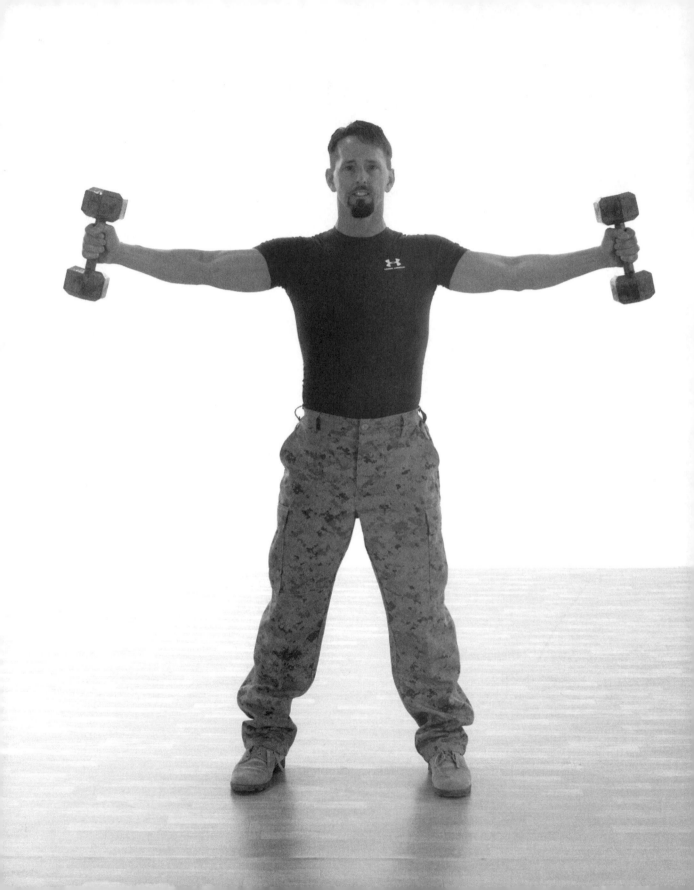

# table of contents

# part 1:
# overview

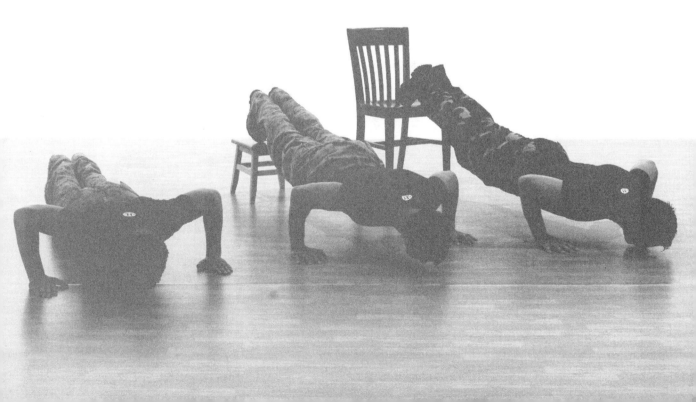

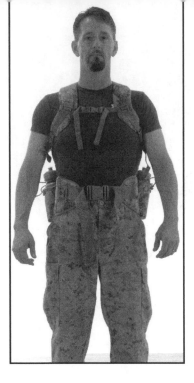

# introduction

When I first started writing fitness books in the 1990s, there were no other manuals based upon the Navy SEAL workout out on the market. Ten years after the first printing, these books are a dime a dozen. Just like any other profession there is progress, growth, and change. I have also learned quite a bit since my first book and decided to bring something unique and different to the market.

For this reason, you will receive nothing but the most informative and effective fitness guidance the market has to offer. Backed by my experience in the fitness industry and military, *Special Ops Fitness Training* will take you to the next level.

In this book, I've taken the best exercises from various Special Forces units to create a program that will generate peak performance. I've also added multiple routines so that your body will never plateau, taking your fitness levels off the charts. The alternative weightlifting program combines calisthenics with free weights to build speed, power, endurance, and size. This book leaves no stone unturned as far as training the upper body, lower body, and abs—you'll also see how the Special Forces include running, swimming, cardio, and weights in their fitness regimens. Whether you're male or female, a beginner or a pro, the exercises and routines in this book will help you achieve results beyond your expectations.

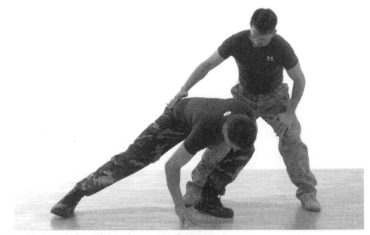

Author Mark De Lisle (right) makes some adjustments.

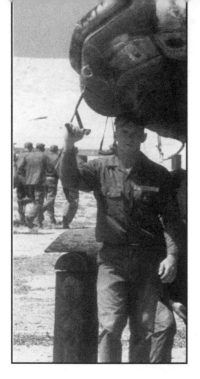

# striving for peak performance

You've probably purchased this book because you're not satisfied with being average—you're looking for something that will take you to the next level of fitness. *Special Ops Fitness Training* will definitely help you get there, but not in the way you might think. The majority of clients I work with are more concerned with how many reps they do rather than performing the exercises correctly. The physical aspect is just a small portion of the peak-performance picture.

In addition, during the training sessions, someone will invariably say, "I can't do any more!" I refuse to let them quit and tell them that they better perform or we're going to be there all day. Take a guess whether they're able to squeeze out those last couple of reps. Sure enough, they do, and they just smile when I remind them that they had nothing left a few reps ago.

Mental domination is essential—you must rise above your body and any weakness in order to function at your peak. Our first reaction while exercising is to listen to our body, and our body's first reaction is to quit under stress. DON'T LISTEN TO IT! From this point forward, you will train like a Special Ops operator and dominate your body so your body can't dominate you. Nobody wants to be a slave to anyone so why let yourself be a slave to your body? It's a weakness, and *Special Ops Fitness Training* eliminates weakness like a bad habit.

Every Special Ops operator has a unique mindset. Failure is not an option so they must find a way to succeed no matter what the cost. You, too, can acquire this mentality by eliminating all doubt from your mind. Not everyone can reach the levels of mental and physical dominance of a Special Ops operator (if anyone could, there wouldn't be anything special about Special Ops), but you can get mighty close. You have to want something so bad that you can taste it, otherwise your motivation will be short-lived. When you begin to feel failure, weakness, or discomfort, take the operator stance and attack it until it becomes a strength. When it comes to your mental strength, take no prisoners and do not look back.

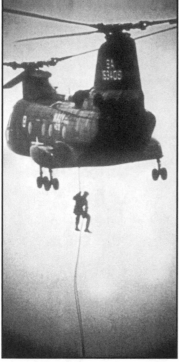

# history of special operations

Modern-day Special Forces can be traced back to Italian assault units, called Arditi, and the German storm trooper of World War II. Both units were specially trained and received extensive training beyond that of the normal infantry; they also had distinct uniforms that separated them from the normal soldiers.

During World War II, British prime minister Winston Churchill formed an elite group of troops known as Special Air Service (SAS), along with the Long Range Desert Group, the Special Boat Service, and the Small Scale Raiding. All were used in unconventional formats, with duties such as reconnaissance, guerrilla tactics, hostage rescue, and assaults.

Many have asked about the difference between U.S. Special Forces and special forces. In most cases, "U.S. Special Forces" refers to Army Green Berets, while the latter refers to all forces within this community. Army or U.S. Special Forces were around as early as World War II, under the direction of Strategic Services; this special group of men performed missions behind enemy lines and gathered intelligence in various locations throughout the world. But the actual origins of modern Special Forces go back a little further.

Major Robert Rogers commanded a unique group of men utilizing unconventional tactics during the French and Indian War. These men enjoyed working in environments that others avoided. Rogers often told his men to "move fast and hit hard." Thanks to these courageous men, later known as Roger's Rangers, the foundation for modern special warfare was laid.

Another pioneer that used the element of surprise to

harass and demoralize the enemy was Francis Marion in the late 18th century. Even though his troop numbers were small, they were very successful on their missions. These units evolved and became the Devil's Brigade, Darby's Rangers, Merrill's Marauders, and Alamo Scouts.

William Donovan, a seasoned veteran of World War I, was able to convince President Franklin D. Roosevelt that a new type of soldier was needed, one who could run secret missions behind enemy lines while collecting intelligence. In 1941 Roosevelt granted Donovan the opportunity to form Coordinator of Intelligence (COI); this organization was soon changed to Office of Strategic Services Society (OSS). In 1952 Special Forces was officially launched.

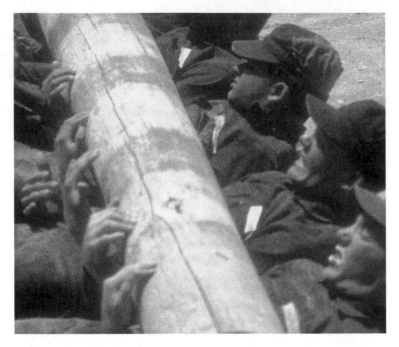

## Air Force Pararescue

*Motto: "That others may live."*

Air Force Special Operations Command has an elite group of men known as Pararescues, or PJs, who are specially equipped to conduct unconventional and conventional rescue operations behind enemy lines or wherever needed. They can perform down-pilot or personnel rescue. These men are incredible combat medics and can handle most situations or injuries they may encounter during a rescue operation. Since they have no idea what they may find in a rescue operation, they have to be on top of all the latest medical skills available, which makes them the most qualified emergency trauma experts in the U.S. military. Because of the need to infiltrate from any scenario, all PJs must be proficient in free-fall sky diving and air operations, as well as skilled in scuba and various other insertion techniques.

The Pararescue unit was purportedly born during World War II, with the China-Burma-India Theater considered the birthplace. Captain John L.

Porter organized the first rescue unit, which flew out of India using two C-47s. Porter's men were able to locate 20 people who had bailed out of a crippled C-46. Having to avoid local Japanese troops and head hunters, they parachuted in one flight surgeon, two combat surgeons, and supplies, while ground troops headed their way. All 20 men were able to find their way out to safety. Realizing a great need for an officially organized command in 1946, Air Rescue Service (ARS) was founded. ARS would eventually change its name to Air Force Pararescue. If you've seen the movie *Air Force One*, Harrison Ford's character was rescued by PJs.

## Army Rangers

*Motto: "Rangers lead the way."*

Army Rangers are a light infantry special operations force based out of Fort Benning, GA. Heeding their motto "Rangers lead the way," they can be deployed anywhere in the world with just an 18-hour notice. This makes them a valuable asset to the Special Forces. The force specializes in airborne; air assaults; light infantry and direct action operations; raids; infiltration and exfiltration by air, land, or sea; airfield seizure; recovery of personnel and special equipment; and support of general purpose forces (GPF). Throughout the decades there have been scenarios where groups of 18 men or less did not provide enough fire or man power to handle the mission. Rangers are trained to work in large numbers while maintaining group integrity and fire superiority, and are also much respected for their reconnaissance and land navigation skills.

The Rangers' origins go back to pre–Revolutionary War days, when colonists surveyed the frontier fortifications, conducting reconnaissance and gathering early warnings of raids from the American Indians. Benjamin Church first organized the group, combining white frontiersman and Indian scouts. His journal was later used as a military manual. During the French and Indian War, Robert Rogers organized a group of New England woodsman to form full-time English auspices (military men) paid under British funds. Roger's Rangers' wilderness skills were so well respected that other military units called upon them for training.

The first group of Army Rangers was hand-picked to perform during World War II. Formed in 1942 as the 1st Ranger Battalion, it began training under Scottish and English commandos. After World War II, the Rangers were disbanded but the training regimen was kept in place, open only to senior non-commissioned officers (NCOs, soldiers who achieved a higher ranking in the military without a college degree) and officers. In 1969, the Rangers were needed in Vietnam and formed into the 75th Ranger Infantry Regiment.

## Green Berets

*Motto: "De Oppresso Liber" (to free the oppressed)*

U.S. Special Forces, or Green Berets, like the Navy SEALs, are generally the first on the ground or at a location when

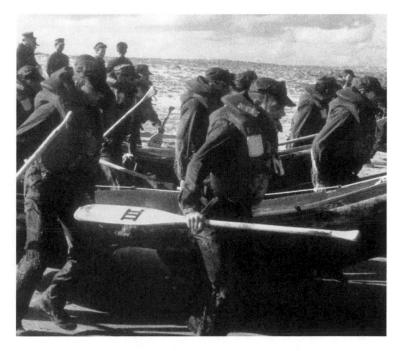

the situation gets hot. Their ability to master foreign languages, customs, and cultures enables them to train foreign troops or insurgents. In order for them to do this, they must be well versed in tactics, weapons, and every facet of war. President John F. Kennedy called Green Berets "a symbol of excellence, a badge of courage, a mark of distinction in the fight for freedom."

Green Berets were officially launched in 1952, evolving from the Coordinator of Intelligence (COI) that World War I veteran William Donovan convinced President Roosevelt to form in 1941. Fort Bragg became the home for Psychological Warfare and Special Forces Center. The

10th Special Forces Group was officially launched with Aaron Bank as their commander. The 10th Special Forces took their ranks from ex-OSS officers, ex-Ranger troops, Airborne, and combat veterans. In 1961 President Kennedy had a unique interest in Special Forces and this led to the adoption of Green Berets.

## Marine Force Recon
*Motto: "Swift, Silent, Deadly."*

Marine Force Recon skills include scout swimming, small boat operations, close-quarter combat (CQB), helicopter and submarine insertion/extraction capabilities, demolition, reconnaissance, and airborne and waterborne insertion missions. Force Recon received its start

in the South Pacific during World War II and was known as Amphibious Reconnaissance Battalion. The Marine Corps merged the Amphibious Reconnaissance Company with an experimental team in 1957 to form 1st Force Reconnaissance Company. Like the SEALs, Force Recon received its first military action during Vietnam, but was deactivated shortly after the conflict ended. The need for Force Recon arose once again in 1986 during the Gulf War. Force Recon has now grown to four units and represents the best of the Marines. Force Recon became an official member of U.S. Special Operations Command in February 2006 and will be a part of the new

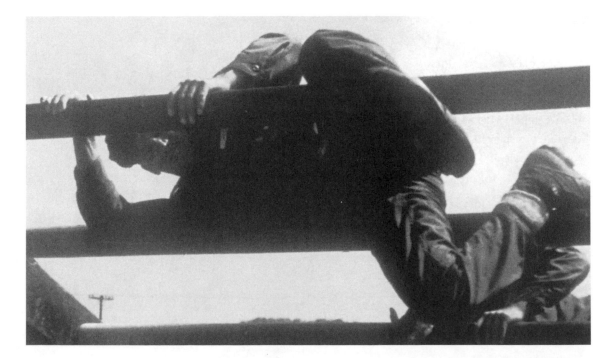

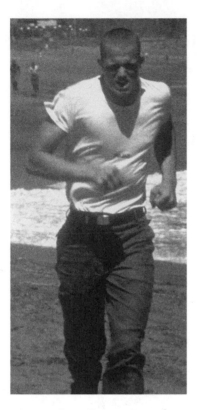

Marine Corp Forces Special Operation Command (MARSOC), which will be fully commissioned by 2010.

### Navy SEALs

*Motto: "The more you sweat in peacetime, the less you bleed in war."*

Navy SEALs (SEAL stands for "sea, air, and land") have the ability to strike from anywhere and at any time. They continue to be a key asset to U.S. Special Operations Command (SOCOM) because they can deploy from ships, submarines, aircraft, helicopters, and small boat operations. Extremely well respected for their clandestine and stealth capabilities, SEALs perform a wide range of special operations. They originally were known only to strike from the sea, but over the years they have proven that their skills are not limited to just the sea. Their versatility is augmented by their skills in small arms, demolition, reconnaissance, unconventional warfare, foreign languages and cultures, and combat martial arts. Their expertise allows them to embark on assault and direct-action missions, as well as engage in close-quarter battle and hostage rescue.

John F. Kennedy saw the direction the world was taking when it came to military struggles and tactics. He envisioned the future would be engaged in more small conflicts rather than larger-scale conflicts. In 1963, he announced that he wanted to form a group that could demoralize and fight the enemy with intense guerilla tactics. Thus the SEALs were formed and received their first opportunity to prove themselves in Vietnam. During the Vietnam War, the SEALs appeared and disappeared in the jungles, which established great fear in the Viet Cong. The SEALs became so feared and respected by their enemies that they were given the nickname "devils with green faces."

Although the SEALs were officially started by President Kennedy, they actually originated during World War II with the Underwater Demolition Teams (UDT), or Frogmen. The UDTs went through some of the most grueling training the military had to offer at that time. During World War II, UDT teams were used to clear beach landing with the demolition they swam in with.

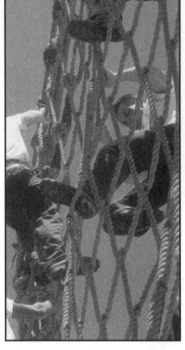

# special ops training

Each branch of the Special Forces has a specialty and each depends on one muscle group more than others. Still, they have to be ready for anything, which requires peak physical conditioning of the entire body. SEALs, for example, need good upper body strength for the amount of swimming they do and possible shipboard attacks; at the same time, if their legs and core are not strong, their swimming will falter.

Marine Force Recon have similar physical needs as the SEALs, and cannot perform and excel if any part of their physical training routine is lacking. Army Rangers and Green Beret are well known for their land capabilities, which demand incredible stamina and leg strength. Yet in an urban arena they could be called upon for anything, so once again they have to be ready. Air Force PJs never know what kind of environment they will encounter due to the wide variety of combat

rescue missions that are found in both non-wartime and wartime campaigns.

To give you a better idea of the excellent shape Special Operations members must be in, this book compiles the minimum physical requirements applicants must meet before they're even considered for recruitment. (You are welcome to visit the following websites for more information: www.bragg.mil, www.specialoperations.com, and www.specialoperations. military.com.) This section also

highlights the mental attitude required to endure the demands and responsibilities of being in the Special Forces and get the job done.

**Air Force Pararescue**
Pararescue undergo some extremely tough and rigorous training, which earns them the right to wear the maroon beret. PJs first must pass a two-week prep course at Lackland Air Force Base in Texas that prepares them to succeed physically in the indoctrination course. Trainees are instructed

in physiological training, dive physics, dive tables, metric manipulations, medical terminology, cardiopulmonary resuscitation, weapons qualifications, PJ history, and leadership reaction. They also engage in obstacle courses and rucksack marches. Afterward, they go through standard EMT training.

Candidates then take a three-week jump school course at Fort Benning. Afterwards, they spend six weeks in Air Force Dive School, where they learn about open- and closed-circuit diving and conduct sub-surface searches and basic recovery missions. A one-day course teaches candidates how to safely escape from a water-bound aircraft. This is followed by a two-and-a-half-week sur-

| PAST Test | | |
|---|---|---|
| **SWIM** | **RUN** | **CALISTHENICS** (with 3-minute breaks in between) |
| • Underwater 20 meters<br>• Rest 5–10 minutes | • 1.5 miles (no maximum time limit)<br>• Rest 10 minutes | • Chin-ups/pull-ups (1 minute) |
| • Surface swim 500 meters using freestyle, breaststroke, or sidestroke<br>• Rest 30 minutes | | • Flutter kicks (2 minutes) |
| | | • Push-ups (2 minutes) |
| | | • Sit-ups (2 minutes) |

## POINTS SCALE FOR PARARESCUE PAST

Note: *You must receive a combined total of 270 points and complete the 20-meter underwater to successfully pass the PAST.*

| SWIM | | RUN | | CALISTHENICS | | | | | |
|---|---|---|---|---|---|---|---|---|---|
| | | | | CHIN-UPS | | Note: *Points are awarded for each area* | | | |
| 500m Time | Points | 1.5-mile Time | Points | Chin-ups Repetitions | Points | Sit-Ups Repetitions | Push-Ups Repetitions | Flutter Kicks Repetitions | Points |
| 16:01 or higher | 10 | 14:01 or higher | 10 | 1 | 3 | 1–5 | 1–5 | 1–5 | 3 |
| 15:41–16:00 | 20 | 13:01–14:00 | 20 | 2 | 5 | 6–10 | 6–10 | 6–10 | 4 |
| 15:21–16:40 | 40 | 12:21–13:00 | 30 | 3 | 7 | 11–15 | 11–15 | 11–15 | 5 |
| 15:01–15:20 | 60 | 12:11–12:20 | 40 | 4 | 10 | 16–20 | 16–20 | 16–20 | 8 |
| 14:41–15:00 | 70 | 12:01–12:10 | 50 | 5 | 15 | 21–25 | 21–25 | 21–25 | 11 |
| 14:21–14:40 | 75 | 11:51–12:00 | 60 | 6 | 20 | 26–30 | 26–30 | 26–30 | 14 |
| 14:01–14:20 | 80 | 11:41–11:50 | 70 | 7 | 23 | 31–35 | 31–35 | 31–35 | 17 |
| 13:41–14:00 | 85 | 11:31–11:40 | 75 | 8 | 25 | 36–40 | 36–40 | 36–40 | 20 |
| 13:21–13:40 | 90 | 11:21–11:30 | 80 | 9 | 26 | 41–45 | 41–45 | 41–45 | 23 |
| 13:01–13:20 | 95 | 11:11–11:20 | 85 | 10 | 27 | 46–50 | 46–50 | 46–50 | 25 |
| 12:01–13:00 | 100 | 11:01–11:10 | 90 | 11 | 28 | 51–55 | 51–55 | 51–55 | 26 |
| 11:01–12:00 | 103 | 10:51–11:00 | 95 | 12 | 29 | 56–60 | 56–60 | 56–60 | 27 |
| 11:00 or below | 105 | 10:31–10:50 | 100 | 13 or more | 30 | 61–65 | 61–65 | 61–65 | 28 |
| | | 10:11–10:30 | 103 | | | 66–70 | 66–70 | 66–70 | 29 |
| | | 10:10 or below | 105 | | | 71 or more | 71 or more | 71 or more | 30 |

vival course. Candidates then attend a five-week free-fall school conducted by the U.S. Army. Pararescue finish their training by attending two very intense medical courses, a 22-week paramedic course and a 24-week Pararescue Recovery Specialist Course.

All candidates must be proficient swimmers and meet specific physical fitness standards as noted in the PAST Test (see page 11).

## Army Rangers

Army Ranger training involves several phases, beginning with a two-week pre-Ranger course to test a candidate's physical and leadership skills and determine whether or not he has what it takes to be a Ranger; Pre-Ranger School also teaches small-unit tactics and land navigation to active and reserve units. Essentially, if you're not already in good physical condition prior to arriving at Ranger School, you'll have a difficult time keeping up.

The Fort Benning Phase incorporates a number of physical challenges. The Army Physical Fitness Test (APFT) requires candidates to do a minimum of 49 push-ups in two minutes, 59 sit-ups in two minutes, and 6 chin-ups. Part of the test includes running five miles, while wearing BDUs

and running shoes, in formation in under 40 minutes; if at any point during the run soldiers fall more than 15 meters behind the formation, they will be considered a run fall-out.

Candidates must also take the Combat Water Survival Test (CWST). The CWST starts with a 15-meter swim while wearing BDUs (camouflage pants), boots, and a load-bearing harness (LBE) with full canteens, and maintaining control of a rubber M16. The test continues in the same uniform; blindfolded, the candidate uses full 30-inch steps until he steps off the diving board and drops three meters into the pool. Once he surfaces, he must confidently swim back to the edge of the pool. In another portion of the test, wearing the same uniform, the candidate steps backward into the pool and releases his rubber M16 and LBE while fully submerged. If the candidate surfaces and any part of the weapon or LBE is still touching his body, this is a "NO-GO." Candidates must receive a "GO" in all events in order to receive a "GO" for CWST.

In addition to the water test, candidates endure a 16-mile foot march along with day and night land navigation courses, and 3-mile runs with an obstacle course. They're also trained

in hand-to-hand combat, basic combat medical skills, terrain association, demolition, and patrol base, and given a refresher parachute jump.

Potential Rangers then move on to Camp William O. Darby in Georgia for their second phase. Here they begin to work on their combat patrol skills in a squad atmosphere. Patrolling skills include boxing, fieldcraft training, Darby Queen obstacle course, communications, and the basics of warning order/operations order format. Ranger candidates must learn battle drills, ambushes, reconnaissance patrols, close-quarters battle (CQB), air operations, and air assault operations. The last step is a final training mission (FTX), where everything is done as realistically as possible.

In the Mountain Phase, adverse weather, rugged terrain, fatigue, and stress challenge Army Ranger candidates mentally, emotionally, and physically. This is where they further develop their survival skills, learn military mountaineering skills, and hone their leadership and soldier skills. They also train how to work with squads and platoons during combat patrol missions in mountainous environments. Candidates must complete a 200-foot night rappel at Yonah Mountain, followed by two FTXs. Over a four-day period, they perform a variety of missions against a conventionally equipped force. They then work as a platoon over a five-day FTX, where they move across the country over mountains, rugged terrain, ambush vehicles, and communications sites using various means such as air assaults or a grueling ten-mile march.

The Final, or Florida, Phase takes place in a jungle or swamp, where candidates work on crossing rivers and streams, as well as other skills necessary for survival in this unique environment. Candidates continue to develop their combat arms skills and leadership abilities; they can also perform a variety of operations, including air, small boat, ship to shore, and dismounted combat control. After a ten-day grueling FTX that incorporates everything they have learned up to that point, they finish their training by parachuting into Fort Benning in an airborne insertion.

## Green Berets

Candidates for Green Beret must score a minimum of 229 points on the Army Physical Fitness Test (APFT), which requires candidates to do a minimum of 49 push-ups in two minutes, 59 sit-ups in two minutes, and 6 chin-ups, as well as run five miles in under forty minutes. They must also be able to meet medical fitness standards. All candidates are given a 50-meter swim assessment, conducted in uniform, during Special Forces Assessment School (SFAS) to determine whether their swimming skills are sufficient to make it through training.

Candidates must first pass a 30-day indoctrination course that allows the Special Forces instructors to ascertain whether or not the soldier has the mental, physical, and emotional stamina to make it through the next phase of training. This also gives the soldier a chance to see if this is truly what he wants. Following this is the Special Forces Qualification Course, which has several phases involving physical training as well as skill acquisition.

Phase One determines a candidate's ability to navigate, operate, and survive in rugged environments day or night. Special skills include land navigation, patrolling, survival air operations, special operations techniques, and small-unit tactics.

Phase Two is geared towards more specialty training, based upon the candidate's unit's needs and the candidate's aptitude toward various skills. There are five categories. SF

Detachment Commander lasts 26 weeks and teaches candidates how to direct and employ other members of his group and best utilize them. SF Weapons Sergeant (24 weeks) educates candidates in all weapons foreign and domestic, weapons tactics, utilization of anti-armor weapons, indirect fire operations, man-portable air-defense weapons, emplacement of weapons, and how to integrate combined-arms fire control. Engineer Sergeant (24 weeks) combines construction and fortification skills along with demolition and explosives. SF Medical Sergeant (57 weeks) provides advanced medical training in the subjects of trauma management and surgical procedures. SF Communications Sergeant (32 weeks) is where candidates learn about radio theory, radio waves, radio communications, and how to apply this in a combat environment.

Phase Three is a culmination of everything candidates have learned up to this point: special operations, air operations, unconventional warfare, and direct action isolation. The phase consists of 38 days in which they integrate and reinforce specialty and common skills training. Candidates are organized into detachments to practice in a realistic environment, where they are hunted

## Marine Corps Physical Fitness Test Points

| Points | Pull-Ups | Crunches (within 2 minutes) | 3-Mile Run | Points | Pull-Ups | Crunches (within 2 minutes) | 3-Mile Run |
|---|---|---|---|---|---|---|---|
| 100 | 20 | 100 | 18:00 | 53 |  | 53 | 25:50 |
| 99 |  | 99 | 18:10 | 52 |  | 52 | 26:00 |
| 98 |  | 98 | 18:20 | 51 |  | 51 | 26:10 |
| 97 |  | 97 | 18:30 | 50 | 10 | 50 | 26:20 |
| 96 |  | 96 | 18:40 | 49 |  | 49 | 26:30 |
| 95 | 19 | 95 | 18:50 | 48 |  | 48 | 26:40 |
| 94 |  | 94 | 19:00 | 47 |  | 47 | 26:50 |
| 93 |  | 93 | 19:10 | 46 |  | 46 | 27:00 |
| 92 |  | 92 | 19:20 | 45 | 9 | 45 | 27:10 |
| 91 |  | 91 | 19:30 | 44 |  | 44 | 27:20 |
| 90 | 18 | 90 | 19:40 | 43 |  | 43 | 27:30 |
| 89 |  | 89 | 19:50 | 42 |  | 42 | 27:40 |
| 88 |  | 88 | 20:00 | 41 |  | 41 | 27:50 |
| 87 |  | 87 | 20:10 | 40 | 8 | 40 | 28:00 |
| 86 |  | 86 | 20:20 | 39 |  | x | 28:10 |
| 85 | 17 | 85 | 20:30 | 38 |  | x | 28:20 |
| 84 |  | 84 | 20:40 | 37 |  | x | 28:30 |
| 83 |  | 83 | 20:50 | 36 |  | x | 28:40 |
| 82 |  | 82 | 21:00 | 35 | 7 | x | 28:50 |
| 81 |  | 81 | 21:10 | 34 |  | x | 29:00 |
| 80 | 16 | 80 | 21:20 | 33 |  | x | 29:10 |
| 79 |  | 79 | 21:30 | 32 |  | x | 29:20 |
| 78 |  | 78 | 21:40 | 31 |  | x | 29:30 |
| 77 |  | 77 | 21:50 | 30 | 6 | x | 29:40 |
| 76 |  | 76 | 22:00 | 29 |  | x | 29:50 |
| 75 | 15 | 75 | 22:10 | 28 |  | x | 30:00 |
| 74 |  | 74 | 22:20 | 27 |  | x | 30:10 |
| 73 |  | 73 | 22:30 | 26 |  | x | 30:20 |
| 72 |  | 72 | 22:40 | 25 | 5 | x | 30:30 |
| 71 |  | 71 | 22:50 | 24 |  | x | 30:40 |
| 70 | 14 | 70 | 23:00 | 23 |  | x | 30:50 |
| 69 |  | 69 | 23:10 | 22 |  | x | 31:00 |
| 68 |  | 68 | 23:20 | 21 |  | x | 31:10 |
| 67 |  | 67 | 23:30 | 20 | 4 | x | 31:20 |
| 66 |  | 66 | 23:40 | 19 |  | x | 31:30 |
| 65 | 13 | 65 | 23:50 | 18 |  | x | 31:40 |
| 64 |  | 64 | 24:00 | 17 |  | x | 31:50 |
| 63 |  | 63 | 24:10 | 16 |  | x | 32:00 |
| 62 |  | 62 | 24:20 | 15 | 3 | x | 32:10 |
| 61 |  | 61 | 24:30 | 14 |  | x | 32:20 |
| 60 | 12 | 60 | 24:40 | 13 |  | x | 32:30 |
| 59 |  | 59 | 24:50 | 12 |  | x | 32:40 |
| 58 |  | 58 | 25:00 | 11 |  | x | 32:50 |
| 57 |  | 57 | 25:10 | 10 |  | x | 33:00 |
| 56 |  | 56 | 25:20 |  |  |  |  |
| 55 | 11 | 55 | 25:30 |  |  |  |  |
| 54 |  | 54 | 25:40 |  |  |  |  |

Round up all values (e.g., 18:01 to 18:09 equals 99 points). 300 points is excellent.

14

and attack live targets to simulate live missions they will encounter as a member of a Special Forces unit.

## Marine Force Recon

After a Marine finishes School of Infantry, he is assigned to an eight-week Basic Recon Course (BRC). Recruits acquire all the skills necessary to operate in a basic reconnaissance environment. Once he has completed BRC, he proceeds to the eight-week Combatant Dive Course, which includes open- and closed-circuit scuba diving, dive laws and physics, underwater searches, and medicine. Upon successful completion of dive school, he advances to Army Airborne Jump School. In this three-week program, new Recon members learn the basics of static line jumping (static line means that the chute automatically opens up as the soldier leaves the plane or helicopter) and get their initial five jumps under their belts. From this point, the Recon can attend many advanced schools such as Freefall, Army Ranger School, Applied Explosives Course, and Helicopter Rope Suspension Training (HRST).

Before soldiers can apply for Marine Force Recon, they must obtain a first-class score (300 points or more) on the Marine Corps Physical Fitness Test (page 14).

## Navy SEALs

SEALs are known to have the toughest military training in the world. What sets the SEALs apart from other military outfits is the fact that their entrance training begins and ends in one place: BUD/S (Basic Underwater Demolition/SEAL School) in San Diego, CA. (Many elite groups receive their training in various locations at various times.) From day one, SEAL wannabes must survive the rigors of acquiring their skills while resisting the on-going pressure from instructors to quit—this creates a scenario where only the best make it through BUD/S. The first phase of training (two months) is very physical, with running, swimming, obstacle courses, physical training (PT) sessions, and daily hammer sessions (wherein instructors push students out of their comfort zones using surf torture, intense exercise, and other team-building drills). SEALs candidates are also introduced to hydro-reconnaissance, stealth, and concealment. It's better known for its infamous Hell Week, when candidates undergo daily training without a wink of sleep. The second phase is the Dive Phase (two months), followed by another two months in the third phase, Land Warfare. Keep in mind that it's not always the strongest and fastest that make it through, but rather the mentally robust. Once the third phase is completed, candidates continue with one month at Parachute Jump School and six

### Navy SEAL Physical Screening Test Requirements

- Swim 500 yards within 12:30 minutes.
- Rest 10 minutes.
- Do 42 push-ups within 2 minutes.
- Rest 2 minutes.
- Do 50 sit-ups within 2 minutes.
- Rest 2 minutes.
- Do 6 pull-ups (no time limit).
- Rest 10 minutes.
- Run 1.5 miles within 11 minutes.

months in advanced sea, air, and land training.

Before they can even be considered for recruitment, Navy SEALs candidates must pass a medical and diving physical examination in addition to completing the Physical Screening Test Requirements.

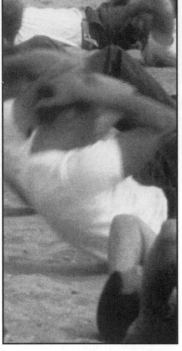

# mental attitude

In this book you'll find everything you need to succeed physically, but there's only one thing that will make you successful with this program—attitude! When any elite soldier's physical abilities have been depleted due to the stresses of training, elements of weather, and intense training schedules, he looks deeply within himself for the necessary motivation—failure is not an option for these individual warriors. No heart, no drive, no desire? Go home.

Similarly, you have to go after your objective like a bull out of the gate. New levels of conditioning, strength, and size don't come easy. You'll have to push yourself hard, but the rewards will be amazing. As you change physically and mentally, you'll acquire higher planes of self-confidence, self-esteem, and drive that will cross over into your relationships and career. You only have one body so take care of it and treat it like a temple—

once it's gone, you can't replace it.

During a cross-training session with some Marines, our assistant officer of Bravo Platoon was getting fired up and ready to go. Then one of the Marine officers said to him, "Stand down, hard charger." That phrase has stuck with me ever since. I don't want you to stand down—I want you to be a hard charger in every aspect, from mental dedication to physical performance to

mental motivation. This is what separates the top notch from the rest. The words "I can't" no longer exist in your vocabulary.

Whether you're a Navy SEAL, Green Beret, Recon, or weekend warrior, you can't live without goals, roadmaps, or motivation. All the motivation in the world won't account for much unless you channel it towards a specific direction or goal. Goals give you a mental destination to focus on while roadmaps show you how to get there. Roadmaps also provide checklists. For example, let's say you want to put on 20 pounds of lean muscle mass. So where do you want to put on this extra weight? Will this require modifying your diet to either gain or lose weight? All this information has to be transferred to paper to make it legit. This checklist covers your diet, exercises (along with reps), and goals, and gives you something to refer to on a daily basis. Nothing brings greater satisfaction than checking off an item on a to-do list. Visual tools such as this are extremely effective in helping you accomplish your goal, so be sure to keep your checklist in a visible place. (You'll find a sample chart on page 20. Make copies to use, or create your own.)

Remember that intelligence plays a major factor in the Special Forces. Physical excellence is just one piece of the puzzle.

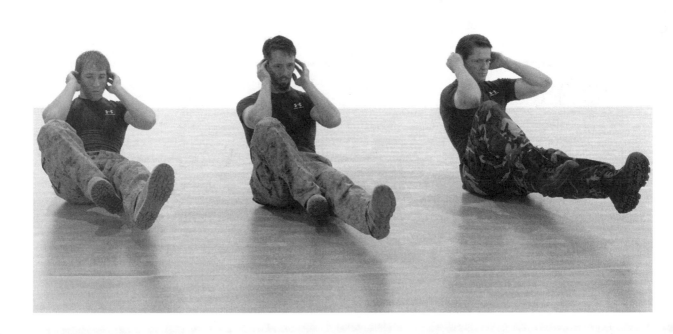

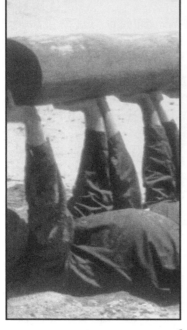

# before you begin

Before you begin any exercise routine, it is recommended you consult a physician. Find out what your limitations are, if any. A doctor most likely will give you the green light, or he may have you modify something based upon your physical conditioning. Either way, don't let ego get in the way of proper exercising. Stepping into this program intelligently allows your body to benefit and develop the way you want it to.

## Equipment

Special Operations incorporate a combination of calisthenics and weight training so that operators have quick-burst strength and energy as well as long-distance or endurance strength that is called upon in many missions. You cannot achieve optimal conditioning with weight training alone; it is not practical and is not always available. In fact, I have operator friends who have never touched weights in their entire lives or stopped after getting into Special Warfare (Spec War). Though numerous soldiers stay in phenomenal shape just by sticking to their own body weight, many say that size and sheer strength cannot be achieved without weights. I know that ever since I strapped on a 50-pound weight vest from weightvest.com and performed push-ups, pull-ups, and dips with it, my training regimens were never the same again.

As far as *Special Ops Fitness Training*, access to a pull-up bar and dip bar is helpful, but you can also use the monkey bars at your local park. You'll just need to be a little creative.

## Injury Prevention

Nothing is more heart wrenching when you're training hard than encountering an injury. In many cases the injury could have been prevented. Although some people say that you don't need to stretch prior to exercising, I disagree and strongly encourage warm-ups and stretching. This does not mean bending over, touching the ground, and saying, "Ahh, that feels good. Let's exercise."

It's important to get the blood flowing into the muscle groups you are going to work, which is where warm-up comes into play. Do not neglect this aspect of your training. Remember, warm up first to get blood flowing into your muscles, then stretch. Your stretching routines should be no less than ten minutes per session.

In many cases there is confusion when it comes to how far you should push yourself when stretching. Whether you're stretching or exercising, there's a distinction between pain and discomfort. Too many people will begin to stretch and stop as soon as they feel just the slightest bit of tightness. The ideal stretch is to go to the point of discomfort, bordering on low-intensity pain, and holding it for a couple of seconds. This discomfort will generally last for ten seconds before it begins to dissipate.

If you have severe lower back pain, consult a doctor to understand the extent of your pain and what your capabilities are. If your lower back is simply tight, however, you will want to stretch out

your calves, hamstrings, and glutes, in addition to your lower back.

When it comes to your joints, it's important to listen to your body. Know when to push it and know when to back off. Once again, do not let your ego get in the way. I have seen people push their bodies too hard because they think they're still 21 years old, or they think that after not working out for a couple of years they can start off right where they left off. So put your ego aside and take things slow. This will be your greatest prevention of injuries that you could ever apply.

Get to know your range of motion. For example, when you're working through your pull-up exercises, go slow in the downward movements. Always remember, when it comes to the speed of exercises, use the same speed going up as the same speed going down. Maintain consistency, whether you've moving forward, back, up, or down.

"Smooth is fast" is what we were taught in the SEAL teams. The reasoning behind it was that when we went too fast, our technique went out the door. So we focused on proper technique and pushed the envelope as hard as we

could, as long as technique was not broken. This same principle would be applied to exercises. There really is no benefit in doing exercises as fast as you can. Your technique will suffer and you're opening yourself up to injury. Remember to consider the range of motion when it comes to your joints. I guarantee that when you perform your exercise at too fast a pace, you will push the limits of your range of motion. Is it worth it to get those extra reps and make the exercise easier yet spend two to six weeks out with torn ligaments?

## The Core of the Matter

The key to a well-conditioned warrior is his core. Without a strong core we are useless. A strong core does not mean only having great upper abs, but rather the upper abs, lower abs, obliques, lower back, and glutes. To achieve optimal conditioning, you must hit every region of your core, from every angle possible. This book includes many kinds of abdominal exercises to provide you with the knowledge base to create your own routines. By changing up these exercises, the intensity, the reps, and the routine, you, too, can achieve a Special Forces core. Take what you have learned here and add it to other routines. The growth is unlimited.

# GOAL & MEASUREMENT CHARTS

Name _____  Body Fat % _____

Start Date _____  Start Weight _____

**Every 30 Days**       Date _____

Neck _____  Shoulders _____  Chest _____

Waist _____  Thigh _____  Calves _____

Weight (Goal)_____  Weight (Current) _____  Body Fat %_____  Body Fat (Current)_____

**Exercise Calisthenics Max**

Pull-Ups (Goal) _____  Pull-Ups _____  Sit-Ups (Goal) _____  Sit-Ups _____

Push-Ups (Goal) _____  Push-Ups _____  Lunges (Goal) _____  Lunges _____

Dips (Goal) _____  Dips _____

**Free-Weight Exercise Max**

Bench (Goal) _____  Bench _____  Curl (Goal) _____  Curl _____

Squat (Goal) _____  Squat _____  Military Press (Goal) _____  Military Press _____

**Every 30 Days**       Date _____

Neck _____  Shoulders _____  Chest _____

Waist _____  Thigh _____  Calves _____

Weight (Goal)_____  Weight (Current) _____  Body Fat %_____  Body Fat (Current)_____

**Exercise Calisthenics Max**

Pull-Ups (Goal) _____  Pull-Ups _____  Sit-Ups (Goal) _____  Sit-Ups _____

Push-Ups (Goal) _____  Push-Ups _____  Lunges (Goal) _____  Lunges _____

Dips (Goal) _____  Dips _____

**Free-Weight Exercise Max**

Bench (Goal) _____  Bench _____  Curl (Goal) _____  Curl _____

Squat (Goal) _____  Squat _____  Military Press (Goal) _____  Military Press _____

# GOAL & MEASUREMENT CHARTS

**Every 30 Days**     Date _____

Neck _____     Shoulders _____     Chest _____

Waist _____     Thigh _____     Calves _____

Weight (Goal)_____ Weight (Current) _____ Body Fat %_____ Body Fat (Current) _____

**Exercise Calisthenics Max**

Pull-Ups (Goal) _____     Pull-Ups _____     Sit-Ups (Goal) _____     Sit-Ups _____

Push-Ups (Goal) _____     Push-Ups _____     Lunges (Goal) _____     Lunges _____

Dips (Goal) _____     Dips _____

**Free-Weight Exercise Max**

Bench (Goal)_____     Bench _____     Curl (Goal) _____     Curl _____

Squat (Goal)_____     Squat_____     Military Press (Goal) _____     Military Press _____

**Every 30 Days**     Date _____

Neck _____     Shoulders _____     Chest _____

Waist _____     Thigh _____     Calves _____

Weight (Goal) _____ Weight (Current) _____ Body Fat % _____ Body Fat (Current) _____

**Exercise Calisthenics Max**

Pull-Ups (Goal) _____     Pull-Ups _____     Sit-Ups (Goal) _____     Sit-Ups _____

Push-Ups (Goal) _____     Push-Ups _____     Lunges (Goal) _____     Lunges _____

Dips (Goal) _____     Dips _____

**Free-Weight Exercise Max**

Bench (Goal)_____     Bench _____     Curl (Goal) _____     Curl _____

Squat (Goal)_____     Squat_____     Military Press (Goal) _____     Military Press _____

# GOAL & MEASUREMENT CHARTS

**Every 30 Days**      Date _____

Neck _____      Shoulders _____      Chest _____

Waist _____      Thigh _____      Calves _____

Weight (Goal)_____ Weight (Current) _____ Body Fat %_____ Body Fat (Current)_____

**Exercise Calisthenics Max**

Pull-Ups (Goal) _____      Pull-Ups _____      Sit-Ups (Goal) _____      Sit-Ups _____

Push-Ups (Goal) _____      Push-Ups _____      Lunges (Goal) _____      Lunges _____

Dips (Goal) _____      Dips _____

**Free-Weight Exercise Max**

Bench (Goal) _____      Bench _____      Curl (Goal) _____      Curl _____

Squat (Goal) _____      Squat _____      Military Press (Goal) _____      Military Press _____

*Before & After Photos*

BEFORE

AFTER

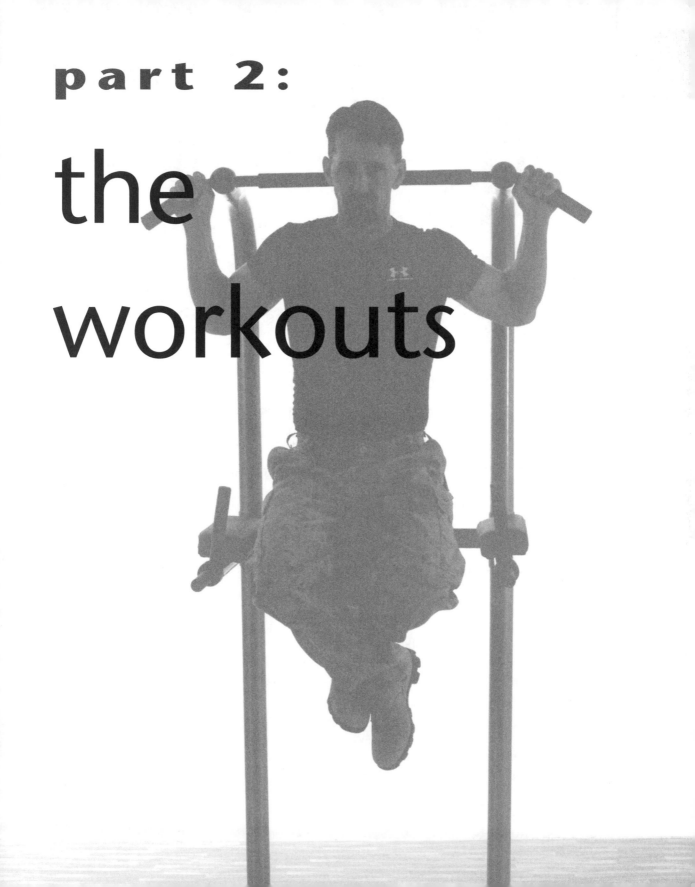

# part 2:
# the
# workouts

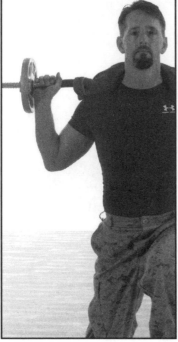

# how to use this book

*Special Ops Fitness Training* will provide you with a complete lifestyle change. The workout routines in this section will help you achieve optimal performance and conditioning, whether you're trying to maintain a certain conditioning level, lose weight, gain muscle, or take your performance to a professional level. Take the routines that I have developed for you and combine them with the workout charts on pages 20–22 to create your own fitness journals.

I recommend performing any of the three Special Ops Routines (pages 28–39) Monday, Wednesday, and Friday for at least 12 solid weeks; the one day of rest in between each workout allows your muscle fibers to build and repair themselves. Each Special Ops Routine takes about 45 to 60 minutes to complete, depending on skill and conditioning. If you don't have that much time in a day

to devote to exercise, you can break up the routines into upper body and lower body sessions and alternate them. In this case, you'd do lower body and abs on Monday, upper body on Tuesday, lower body and abs on Wednesday, upper body on Thursday, lower body and abs on Friday, and upper body on Saturday. In addition to doing these routines on their own, you can also combine them with other exercises

or incorporate the appropriate Alternative Workout (pages 50–52).

After at least 12 weeks, you can break up the program by utilizing any of the five individual branch programs. Switching up the routines you do will make it very difficult for your body to plateau, which means it can only get stronger in order to keep up with your demands.

Focusing is a major factor in peak performance. Many times I'll watch a client work out and catch him looking off in one direction then another—right in the middle of his rep. That same person then attempts to complete six pull-ups but wants to quit at number four. That's when I make him choose a spot on the wall or ceiling, depending on the position of his body. He takes that spot and looks at it like a site on a gun. When he sees that object in perfect focus and everything else goes blurry, he's ready to perform his exercise. Try it—the difference it makes in your training will be significant.

## Stretching

Stretching is one of the most neglected categories in any exercise routine. Whether you're a Navy SEAL, Green Beret, Army Ranger, Recon, or PJ, you will need incredible flexibility so make sure to stretch after every workout and take your time. This does not mean getting into position, going to the point of discomfort, and then releasing it. The key to stretching is to go to the point of discomfort then wait until that discomfort dissipates. Proper breathing is another important part of stretching. Once you reach the point of discomfort, take a deep breath and exhale slowly and audibly; try to relax every fiber in the muscle you are stretching. Another key point to effective stretching is not to

bounce. This does not help you to get the most out of your stretch routine; in some cases it can even cause injury.

Increase the effectiveness of your stretching routine by spending a good five to ten minutes doing so at the end of your routine. Remember that your greatest gains in flexibility occur post-workout. You might also consider spending 60 to 90 seconds stretching the specific muscles you just worked out. For example, if I'm performing push-ups, I'll do chest stretches after the third set or at the peak of my pyramid. I seem to be able to push myself a little harder afterwards while alleviating the stress on the muscle at the same time.

Abdominal stretches should be performed every third abs exercise. This helps prevent the muscles in your stomach from tightening up. Perform the Cobra Stretch (page 75) when exercising your upper, middle, and oblique muscles. Lower Back Stretch (page 78) is excellent for loosening up your lower back; it can also be used to alleviate lower back strain if you enlist a partner to help you stretch.

When it comes to your back, always take extra care. I have been in two major car accidents. Add to that the

stresses that Special Ops can play on your body and my back can act up. If it were not for these exercises and stretches I could be in a lot of pain. I have also noticed that if I back off of my training for a certain period of time, my back can act up. Therefore, if you have back problems, seek permission from your doctor before performing these exercises. Once again, take your

## TAKING IT OUTSIDE

If you want to apply physical fitness in a more practical environment or if you wish to help your body adapt to the rigors of a Special Ops mission, then find a local park that has monkey bars, an obstacle course, a ropes course, or a physical fitness course. This kind of equipment will allow your body to experience muscle exertion under higher stress levels. There's nothing like running a mile and then performing push-ups and pull-ups, or maneuvering a monkey bar. If you come across a log while doing a long-distance run, increase your hand-eye coordination by running down it. Hopping over obstacles and hurdles can greatly enhance your quick-burst muscle. When it comes down to it, you must be well-rounded if you expect to succeed. If you want to train like the Special Forces, then train for the unexpected.

## VISUALIZATION

Sometimes if you have difficulty getting your muscles to exercise and perform at their optimum level, try visualizing. For example, when I perform a Behind-the-Neck Pull-Up, I picture just my inner back and back muscles working. I visualize perfect form before and while I do my exercise. You'll soon see improvement in your technique.

time when it comes to stretching and take advantage of the lower back stretch.

## Special Ops Exercises & Free Weights

Navy SEALs have always joked about heavy body builders as having useless muscles. If you're going to incorporate weights into your routine, then be smart about it and create useful muscles. It means nothing if you have incredible strength for 30 to 60 seconds. I want you to have incredible strength that will last for 30 minutes to whatever it takes to get the job done. That's why I've included the Alternative Workout (pages 50–52).

To get the most out of your weigh training while maximizing your calisthenics, I've laid out a complete routine that combines the best calisthenics and free weights exercise for

optimum results. It's generally best to do a related calisthenics exercises at the end of your weights exercises. For example, start on a flat bench to work the chest and triceps. Next, move on to butterflies with either dumbbells or the butterfly machine. Your chest is now primed to maximize a push-up routine (the calisthenics).

### Routine Cycling

No matter what kind of shape you're in and regardless of how successful your existing exercise program may be, your body's natural reaction to any intense training program is to get bored over a certain period of time and plateau, adjusting to the workload and making it easier to perform. Your body is an amazing instrument, and it's smart. It has a survival mechanism and its first priority is to protect itself from stress and strain. For this reason, I lay out the Alternative Workout routine over a three-day period. The example below shows which body parts to

work each week. Unlike calisthenics, which require one day of rest, weightlifting routines need two to three days' rest between body parts.

By rotating your workout patterns, *Special Ops Fitness Training* creates an environment in which you're able to confuse your body and keep it in a state of shock. Take this book and grow, adapt, and expand. This may be the greatest exercise routine you've ever experienced.

### Pyramid & Burnout

For about six weeks, perform the routines as laid out. The next six weeks, you may pyramid: for instance, doing 4 reps/rest/6 reps/rest/8 reps/rest/6 reps/rest/4 reps. You may start to peak as the reps get higher; this is when you should reduce the number of reps, which helps you keep good form as your body gets tired.

Before your body gets used to the pyramid, perhaps the week after, you might incorpo-

| WEEK ONE | |
|---|---|
| **MONDAY** | Chest / Triceps |
| **TUESDAY** | Legs / Biceps |
| **WEDNESDAY** | Shoulders / Back |
| **THURSDAY** | Chest / Triceps |
| **FRIDAY** | Legs / Biceps |

| WEEK TWO | |
|---|---|
| **MONDAY** | Shoulders / Back |
| **TUESDAY** | Chest / Triceps |
| **WEDNESDAY** | Legs / Biceps |
| **THURSDAY** | Shoulders / Back |
| **FRIDAY** | Chest / Triceps |

rate burnouts, where you go as hard as you can for as long as you can during one exercise. When you have nothing left, switch to the next exercise and burn out on this one. Burnout won't take as long as other routines but they leave you even more exhausted. Never perform burnouts over an extended period of time. If you do need to perform burnouts, do them several days in a row but then go back to another routine. You don't want to make yourself prone to injury. Burnouts have a tendency to stress the muscle groups dramatically and you'll need a certain period of time to repair.

As you can see, there are many ways to keep the body guessing. With this manual, you'll have sufficient routines and exercises to keep you going for a very long time.

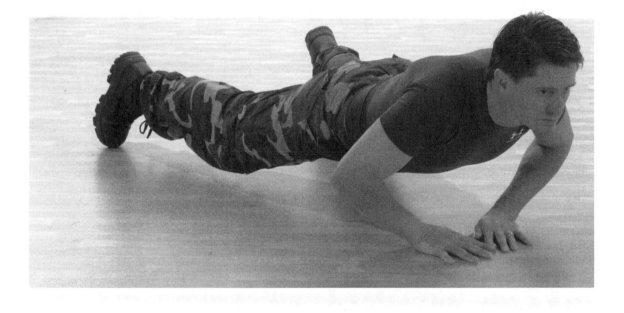

## SPECIAL OPS ROUTINE 1

| | p. 56 | Jumping Jacks | 1 x 30 secs |
|---|---|---|---|
| | p. 57 | Half Jumping Jacks | 1 x 30 secs |
| | p. 58 | Iron Mikes | 1 x 30 secs |
| | p. 65 | V Stretch | 1 x 30 secs |
| | p. 60 | Upper Back Stretch | 1 x 30 secs |
| | p. 78 | Partner-Assisted Lower Back Stretch | 1 x 30 secs each side |
| | p. 68 | Hamstring Stretch | 1 x 30 secs |
| | p. 69 | Trunk Stretch | 1 x 30 secs each side |
| | p. 70 | Groin Stretch | 1 x 30 secs each side |
| | p. 72 | Quad Stretch | 1 x 30 secs each side |
| | p. 66 | Straight-Leg Stretch | 1 x 30 secs |
| | p. 67 | ITB Stretch | 1 x 30 secs each side |
| | p. 62 | Tricep Stretch | 1 x 30 secs each side |
| | p. 61 | Forearm Stretch | 1 x 30 secs each side |

# SPECIAL OPS ROUTINE 1

## STRETCHES

| | | | |
|---|---|---|---|
| | p. 71 | Partner Butterfly | 1 x 30 secs |
| | p. 73 | Calf Stretch #1 | 1 x 30 secs each side |
| | p. 75 | Cobra Stretch | 1 x 30 secs |
| | p. 76 | Cat Back Stretch | 1 x 30 secs |
| | p. 59 | Chest Stretch | 1 x 30 secs each side |
| | p. 63 | Partner-Assisted Upper Body Stretch | 1 x 30 secs |
| | p. 64 | Side-to-Side Stretch | 1 x 30 secs each side |

## UPPER BODY

| | | | |
|---|---|---|---|
| | p. 80 | Pull-Up: Regular | *Set 1:* max reps/*Set 2:* 75% of last set/ *Set 3:* 75% of last set/*Set 4:* 75% of last set |
| | p. 83 | Pull-Up: Behind the Neck | *Set 1:* max reps/*Set 2:* 75% of last set/ *Set 3:* 75% of last set/*Set 4:* 75% of last set |
| | p. 84 | Dip | *Set 1:* max reps/*Set 2:* 75% of last set/ *Set 3:* 75% of last set/*Set 4:* 75% of last set |
| | p. 85 | Push-Up: Regular | *Set 1:* max reps/*Set 2:* 75% of last set/ *Set 3:* 75% of last set/*Set 4:* 75% of last set |
| | p. 86 | Push-Up: Diamond | *Set 1:* max reps/*Set 2:* 75% of last set/ *Set 3:* 75% of last set/*Set 4:* 75% of last set |
| | p. 87 | Push-Up: Ranger Diamond | *Set 1:* max reps/*Set 2:* 75% of last set/ *Set 3:* 75% of last set/*Set 4:* 75% of last set |
| | p. 88 | Push-Up: Triple Sets | *Set 1:* max reps/*Set 2:* 75% of last set/ *Set 3:* 75% of last set/*Set 4:* 75% of last set |

# SPECIAL OPS ROUTINE 1

| | p. 90 | Push-Up: Elevated | max reps at each position |
|---|---|---|---|
| | p. 85 | (Optional) Partner-Assisted Push-Up | 4 x max reps |

| | p. 92 | Eight-Count Body Builders | *Set 1:* 60 secs/*Set 2:* 45 secs/ *Set 3:* 30 secs/*Set 4:* 15 secs |
|---|---|---|---|
| | p. 94 | Walking Lunge | *Set 1:* 50 yards at medium pace (timed)/ *Set 2:* 50 yards 15 secs faster/*Set 3:* 50 yards 10 secs faster |
| | p. 97 | Wall Sit | 10 minutes |
| | p. 95 | Frog Hop | 3 x 50 yards |
| | p. 96 | Star Hop | 3 x 20 reps |
| | p. 102 | Ruck Sack March (to be done after leg routine or abs workout) | 6 miles |

| | p. 116 | Fly My Airplane | *Set 1:* 60 secs/*Set 2:* 45 secs/*Set 3:* 30 secs |
|---|---|---|---|
| | p. 101 | Bench Back Exercise | *Set 1:* 60 secs/*Set 2:* 45 secs/*Set 3:* 30 secs |
| | p. 104 | Hand to Toes | 1 x 60 reps |
| | p. 106 | Ranger Crunch | 1 x 60 reps |
| | p. 105 | X Sit-Up | 1 x 60 reps |
| | p. 107 | Supine Bicycle | 1 x 60 reps |

# SPECIAL OPS ROUTINE 1

**ABDOMINALS**

| | p.108 | Hibberty Jibberty | 1 x 60 reps |
|---|---|---|---|
| | p. 109 | Cross Crunch | 1 x 60 reps |
| | p. 112 | Sky Hop | 1 x 60 reps |
| | p. 111 | Flutter Kick | 1 x 60 reps |
| | p. 113 | Lower Ab Crunch | 1 x 60 reps |
| | p. 114 | Scissor Lift | 1 x 60 reps |
| | p. 115 | (Optional) Bench Sit-Up | 1 x 60 reps |

# SPECIAL OPS ROUTINE 2

**WARM-UP**

| | p. 56 | Jumping Jacks | 1 x 30 secs |
|---|---|---|---|
| | p. 57 | Half Jumping Jacks | 1 x 30 secs |
| | p. 58 | Iron Mikes | 1 x 30 secs |

**STRETCHES**

| | p. 65 | V Stretch | 1 x 30 secs each side |
|---|---|---|---|
| | p. 60 | Upper Back Stretch | 1 x 30 secs |
| | p. 77 | Partner-Assisted Lower Back Twist | 1 x 30 secs each side |
| | p. 68 | Hamstring Stretch | 1 x 30 secs |
| | p. 69 | Trunk Stretch | 1 x 30 secs each side |
| | p. 70 | Groin Stretch | 1 x 30 secs each side |
| | p. 72 | Quad Stretch | 1 x 30 secs each side |
| | p. 66 | Straight-Leg Stretch | 1 x 30 secs |
| | p. 67 | ITB Stretch | 1 x 30 secs each side |
| | p. 62 | Tricep Stretch | 1 x 30 secs each side |
| | p. 61 | Forearm Stretch | 1 x 30 secs each side |

# SPECIAL OPS ROUTINE 2

## STRETCHES

| | p. 71 | Partner Butterfly | 1 x 30 secs |
|---|---|---|---|
| | p. 74 | Calf Stretch #2 | 1 x 30 secs each side |
| | p. 75 | Cobra Stretch | 1 x 30 secs |
| | p. 76 | Cat Back Stretch | 1 x 30 secs |
| | p. 63 | Partner-Assisted Chest Stretch | 1 x 30 secs each side |
| | p. 63 | Partner-Assisted Upper Body Stretch | 1 x 30 secs |
| | p. 64 | Side-to-Side Stretch | 1 x 30 secs each side |

## UPPER BODY

| | p. 80 | Pull-Up: Regular | 8–10–12–14–16–14–12–10–8 |
|---|---|---|---|
| | p. 83 | Pull-Up: Behind the Neck | 4–6–8–10–8–6–4 |
| | p. 84 | Dip | 4 x 25 reps |
| | p. 85 | Push-Up: Regular | 12–14–16–18–20–22–24–26–24–22–20–18–16–14–12 |
| | p. 86 | Push-Up: Diamond | 8–10–12–14–16–14–12–10–8 |
| | p. 87 | Push-Up: Ranger Diamond | 4 x 10 reps |
| | p. 88 | Push-Up: Triple Sets | 4 x 20 wide, 15 regular, 10 diamond |

# SPECIAL OPS ROUTINE 2

| | | | |
|---|---|---|---|
| **UPPER** | p. 90 | Push-Up: Elevated | *Position 1:* 20 reps/*Position 2:* 25 reps/ *Position 3:* 30 reps |
| | p. 85 | (Optional) Partner-Assisted Push-Up | *Set 1:* 60 secs/*Set 2:* 45 secs/ *Set 3:* 30 secs/*Set 4:* 15 secs |
| **LOWER BODY** | p. 92 | Eight-Count Body Builders | *Set 1:* 20 reps/*Set 2:* 15 reps/ *Set 3:* 10 reps/*Set 4:* 5 reps |
| | p. 94 | Walking Lunge | *Set 1:* 50 yards 40 lbs/*Set 2:* 50 yards 30 lbs/ *Set 3:* 50 yards 20 lbs |
| | p. 97 | Wall Sit | 10 minutes |
| | p. 95 | Frog Hop | 3 x 50 yards |
| | p. 96 | Star Hop | 3 x 20 reps |
| | p. 102 | Ruck Sack March (to be performed after your leg routine or abs workout) | 6 miles |
| **ABDOMINALS** | p. 116 | Fly My Airplane | *Set 1:* 60 secs/*Set 2:* 45 secs/ *Set 3:* 30 secs |
| | p. 101 | Bench Back Exercise | *Set 1:* 60 secs/*Set 2:* 45 secs/ *Set 3:* 30 secs |
| | p. 104 | Hand to Toes | 1 x 60 reps |
| | p. 106 | Ranger Crunch | 1 x 60 reps |
| | p. 105 | X Sit-Up | 1 x 60 reps |
| | p. 107 | Supine Bicycle | 1 x 60 reps |

# SPECIAL OPS ROUTINE 2

| | | | |
|---|---|---|---|
| | p. 108 | Hibberty Jibberty | 1 x 60 reps |
| | p. 109 | Cross Crunch | 1 x 60 reps |
| | p. 112 | Sky Hop | 1 x 60 reps |
| | p. 111 | Flutter Kick | 1 x 60 reps |
| | p. 113 | Lower Ab Crunch | 1 x 60 reps |
| | p. 114 | Scissor Lift | 1 x 60 reps |
| | p. 115 | (Optional) Bench Sit-Up | 1 x 60 reps |

ABDOMINALS

# SPECIAL OPS ROUTINE 3

## WARM-UP

| | p. 56 | Jumping Jacks | 1 x 30 secs |
|---|---|---|---|
| | p. 57 | Half Jumping Jacks | 1 x 30 secs |
| | p. 58 | Iron Mikes | 1 x 30 secs |

## STRETCHES

| | p. 65 | V Stretch | 1 x 30 secs each side |
|---|---|---|---|
| | p. 60 | Upper Back Stretch | 1 x 30 secs |
| | p. 78 | Partner-Assisted Lower Back Stretch | 1 x 30 secs each side |
| | p. 68 | Hamstring Stretch | 1 x 30 secs |
| | p. 69 | Trunk Stretch | 1 x 30 secs each side |
| | p. 70 | Groin Stretch | 1 x 30 secs each side |
| | p. 72 | Quad Stretch | 1 x 30 secs each side |
| | p. 66 | Straight-Leg Stretch | 1 x 30 secs |
| | p. 67 | ITB Stretch | 1 x 30 secs each side |
| | p. 62 | Tricep Stretch | 1 x 30 secs each side |
| | p. 61 | Forearm Stretch | 1 x 30 secs each side |

# SPECIAL OPS ROUTINE 3

**STRETCHES**

| | p. 71 | Partner Butterfly | 1 x 30 secs |
|---|---|---|---|
| | p. 73 | Calf Stretch #1 | 1 x 30 secs each side |
| | p. 75 | Cobra Stretch | 1 x 30 secs |
| | p. 76 | Cat Back Stretch | 1 x 30 secs |
| | p. 59 | Chest Stretch | 1 x 30 secs each side |
| | p. 63 | Partner-Assisted Upper Body Stretch | 1 x 30 secs |
| | p. 64 | Side-to-Side Stretch | 1 x 30 secs each side |

**UPPER BODY**

| | p. 80 | Pull-Up: Regular | *Set 1:* 60 secs/*Set 2:* 45 secs/ *Set 3:* 30 secs/*Set 4:* 15 secs (contraction) |
|---|---|---|---|
| | p. 83 | Pull-Up: Behind the Neck | *Set 1:* 60 secs/*Set 2:* 45 secs/ *Set 3:* 30 secs/*Set 4:* 15 secs (contraction) |
| | p. 84 | Dip | *Set 1:* 60 secs/*Set 2:* 45 secs/ *Set 3:* 30 secs/*Set 4:* 15 secs (contraction) |
| | p. 85 | Push-Up: Regular | *Set 1:* 60 secs/*Set 2:* 45 secs/ *Set 3:* 30 secs/*Set 4:* 15 secs (contraction) |
| | p. 86 | Push-Up: Diamond | *Set 1:* 60 secs/*Set 2:* 45 secs/ *Set 3:* 30 secs/*Set 4:* 15 secs (contraction) |
| | p. 87 | Push-Up: Ranger Diamond | *Set 1:* 60 secs/*Set 2:* 45 secs/ *Set 3:* 30 secs/*Set 4:* 15 secs (contraction) |
| | p. 88 | Push-Up: Triple Sets | *Sets 1–3:* 20 secs wide, 15 secs regular/10 secs diamond/ *Set 4:* same as Sets 1–3, but all with contraction |

## SPECIAL OPS ROUTINE 3

**UPPER**

| | p. 90 | Push-Up: Elevated | *Position 1:* 60 secs/*Position 2:* 45 secs/ *Position 3:* 30 secs |
|---|---|---|---|
| | p.85 | (Optional) Partner-Assisted Push-Up | *Set 1:* 60 secs/*Set 2:* 45 secs/ *Set 3:* 30 secs |

**LOWER BODY**

| | p. 92 | Eight-Count Body Builders | *Set 1:* 60 secs/*Set 2:* 45 secs/ *Set 3:* 30 secs/*Set 4:* 15 secs |
|---|---|---|---|
| | p. 94 | Walking Lunge | *Set 1:* 50 yards medium pace (timed)/ *Set 2:* 50 yards 15 secs faster/*Set 3:* 50 yards 10 secs faster |
| | p. 97 | Wall Sit | 10 minutes |
| | p. 95 | Frog Hop | *Set 1:* 60 secs/*Set 2:* 45 secs/ *Set 3:* 30 secs |
| | p. 96 | Star Hop | *Set 1:* 45 secs/*Set 2:* 30 secs/ *Set 3:* 15 secs |
| | p. 102 | Ruck Sack March (to be performed after your leg routine or abs workout) | 6 miles |

**ABDOMINALS**

| | p. 116 | Fly My Airplane | *Set 1:* 60 secs/*Set 2:* 45 secs/ *Set 3:* 30 secs |
|---|---|---|---|
| | p. 101 | Bench Back Exercise | *Set 1:* 60 secs/*Set 2:* 45 secs/ *Set 3:* 30 secs |
| | p. 104 | Hand to Toes | 1 x 60 secs |
| | p. 106 | Ranger Crunch | 1 x 60 secs |
| | p. 105 | X Sit-Up | 1 x 60 secs |
| | p. 107 | Supine Bicycle | 1 x 60 secs |

# SPECIAL OPS ROUTINE 3

| | | | |
|---|---|---|---|
| | p. 108 | Hibberty Jibberty | 1 x 60 secs |
| | p. 109 | Cross Crunch | 1 x 60 secs |
| | p. 112 | Sky Hop | 1 x 60 secs |
| | p. 111 | Flutter Kick | 1 x 60 secs |
| | p. 113 | Lower Ab Crunch | 1 x 60 secs |
| | p. 114 | Scissor Lift | 1 x 60 secs |
| | p. 115 | (Optional) Bench Sit-Up | 1 x 60 secs |

# AIR FORCE PARARESCUE

*Air Force PJs may be required to haul their objective out of enemy territory. This requires excellent upper body strength and good leg endurance for the long haul. At the same time, PJs require a lot of quick-burst muscles to get in and out fast.*

| | | | |
|---|---|---|---|
| | p. 56 | Jumping Jacks | 1 x 60 secs |
| | p. 57 | Half Jumping Jacks | 1 x 60 secs |
| | pp. 59–79 | Stretches | 1 x 30 secs each |
| | p. 80 | Pull-Up: Regular | *Set 1:* 60 secs/*Set 2:* 45 secs/ *Set 3:* 30 secs/*Set 4:* 15 secs |
| | p. 84 | Dip | 4 x 25 reps |
| | p. 85 | Push-Up: Regular | *Set 1:* 100 reps/*Set 2:* 30 secs burn-out/ *Set 3:* 20 (4 count) |
| | p. 86 | Push-Up: Diamond | *Set 1:* 30 reps/*Set 2:* 30 secs burn-out/ *Set 3:* 15 (4 count) |
| | p. 88 | Push-Up: Triple Sets | 30 secs burn-out at each position |
| | p. 94 | Walking Lunges | 4 x 45 secs as fast as you can |

**CARDIO**
- Monday 3-mile run
- Wednesday 1-mile swim (freestyle)
- Friday 3-mile run

# AIR FORCE PARARESCUE

**The following are all performed in burn-out mode—as many as you can in 30 seconds**

| | p. 104 | Hand to Toes | 1 x 30 secs |
|---|---|---|---|
| | p. 105 | X Sit-Up | 1 x 30 secs |
| | p. 108 | Hibberty Jibberty | 1 x 30 secs |
| | p. 109 | Cross Crunch | 1 x 30 secs |
| | p. 110 | Obliques | 1 x 30 secs |
| | p. 112 | Sky Hop | 1 x 30 secs |
| | p. 113 | Lower Ab Crunch | 1 x 30 secs |
| | p. 114 | Scissor Lift | 1 x 30 secs |
| | p. 111 | Flutter Kick | 1 x 30 secs |

# ARMY RANGER

*Of all the Special Forces, Army Rangers require the highest level of endurance due to their missions involving deep enemy territory penetration. They must have high levels of strength in all parts of their body, but especially in their legs.*

| | | | |
|---|---|---|---|
| | p. 56 | Jumping Jacks | 1 x 60 secs |
| | p. 58 | Iron Mikes | 1 x 60 secs |
| | pp 59–79 | Stretches | 1 x 30 secs each |
| | p. 80 | Pull-Up: Regular | *Set 1:* 10 reps/*Set 2:* 8 reps/ *Set 3:* 6 reps/*Set 4:* 4 reps |
| | p. 84 | Dip | *Set 1:* 25 reps/*Set 2:* 20 reps/ *Set 3:* 15 reps/*Set 4:* 10 reps |
| | p. 85 | Push-Up: Regular | 4 x 20 reps (4 count) |
| | p. 87 | Push-Up: Ranger Diamond | 4 x 20 reps |
| | p. 92 | Eight-Count Body Builders | 4 x 90 secs |
| | p. 94 | Walking Lunge | 4 x 90 secs |
| CARDIO | • Monday 10-mile Ruck Sack March • Wednesday 3-mile run • Friday 15-mile Ruck Sack March | | |

# ARMY RANGER

**The following are all performed in a controlled pace—
do as many as you can with perfect technique.**

| | | | |
|---|---|---|---|
| | p. 105 | X Sit-Up | 1 x 60 secs |
| | p. 106 | Ranger Crunch | 1 x 60 secs |
| | p. 108 | Hibberty Jibberty | 1 x 60 secs |
| | p. 109 | Cross Crunch | 1 x 60 secs |
| | p. 112 | Sky Hop | 1 x 60 secs |
| | p. 113 | Lower Ab Crunch | 1 x 60 secs |
| | p. 114 | Scissor Lift | 1 x 60 secs |

ARMY RANGER

# GREEN BERET

*Green Beret/Delta Force require high levels of strength and endurance.*

| | | | |
|---|---|---|---|
| | p. 56 | Jumping Jacks | 1 x 60 secs |
| | p. 58 | Iron Mikes | 1 x 60 secs |
| | pp 59–79 | Stretches | 1 x 30 secs each |
| | p. 80 | Pull-Up: Regular | *Set 1:* Burn-out/*Sets 2–7:* 8 reps |
| | p. 84 | Dip | 4 x 15 reps |
| | p. 85 | Push-Up: Regular | 1 x 20 reps (5 count) |
| | p. 87 | Push-Up: Ranger Diamond | 4 x 20 reps |
| | p. 88 | Push-Up: Triple Sets | 1 x 20 reps |
| | p. 92 | Eight-Count Body Builders | 1 x 30 reps |
| | p. 94 | Lunges (Standing—step left, step right = 1 rep) | 1 x 100 reps |

| CARDIO | • Monday 3-mile run<br>• Wednesday 15-mile Ruck Sack March<br>• Friday 3-mile run |
|---|---|

# GREEN BERET

**The following are performed with 20 seconds of rest in between each set.**

| | | | |
|---|---|---|---|
| | p. 104 | Hand to Toes | 1 x 65 reps |
| | p. 106 | Ranger Crunch | 1 x 65 reps |
| | p. 108 | Hibberty Jibberty | 1 x 65 reps |
| | p. 109 | Cross Crunch | 1 x 65 reps |
| | p. 112 | Sky Hop | 1 x 65 reps |
| | p. 113 | Lower Ab Crunch | 1 x 65 reps |
| | p. 114 | Scissor Lift | 1 x 65 reps |

# MARINE FORCE RECON

*The operators in Marine Special Forces units (Marine Special Operations Command, or MARSOC) have similar requirements as SEALs.*

| | | | |
|---|---|---|---|
| | p. 56 | Jumping Jacks | 1 x 60 secs |
| | p. 57 | Half Jumping Jacks | 1 x 60 secs |
| | pp. 59–79 | Stretches | 1 x 30 secs each |
| | p. 80 | Pull-Up: Regular | *Set 1:* 30 reps/*Set 2:* 25 reps/ *Set 3:* 20 reps/*Set 4:* 15 reps |
| | p. 82 | Pull-Up: Close Grip | *Set 1:* 20 reps/*Set 2:* 15 reps/*Set 3:* 10 reps |
| | p. 83 | Pull-Up: Behind the Neck | *Set 1:* 15 reps/*Set 2:* 10 reps/*Set 3:* 5 reps |
| | p. 84 | Dip | 4 x 25 reps |
| | p. 85 | Push-Up: Regular | *Set 1:* 100 reps/*Set 2:* 75 reps/ *Set 3:* 50 reps/*Set 4:* 25 reps |
| | p. 86 | Push-Up: Diamond | *Set 1:* 25 reps/*Set 2:* 20 reps/ *Set 3:* 15 reps/*Set 4:* 10 reps |
| | p. 92 | Eight-Count Body Builders | 4 x 15 reps |
| | p. 94 | Walking Lunge | 4 x 50 yards |

| CARDIO | • Monday 3-mile run<br>  • Wednesday 1-mile swim (freestyle)<br>    • Friday 1-mile interval sprints (sprint on straightaway and jog the corners) |
|---|---|

# MARINE FORCE RECON

| | | | |
|---|---|---|---|
| | p. 104 | Hand to Toes | 1 x 65 reps |
| | p. 105 | X Sit-Up | 1 x 65 reps |
| | p. 106 | Ranger Crunch | 1 x 65 reps |
| | p.108 | Hibberty Jibberty | 1 x 65 reps |
| | p.110 | Obliques | 1 x 65 reps |
| | p. 113 | Lower Ab Crunch | 1 x 65 reps |
| | p. 111 | Flutter Kicks | 1 x 45 reps (4 count) |

# NAVY SEAL

*SEALs need quick-burst energy but sometimes have to swim up to three hours at a time. High levels of upper body strength could be needed at any given moment. Combine this workout with the other workouts provided in this book and there is no excuse for not being ready physically for BUD/S.*

| | p. 56 | Jumping Jacks | 1 x 60 secs |
|---|---|---|---|
| | p. 57 | Half Jumping Jacks | 1 x 60 secs |
| | pp. 59–79 | Stretches | 1 x 30 secs each |
| | p. 80 | Pull-Up: Regular | *Set 1:* 30 reps/*Set 2:* 25 reps/*Set 3:* 20 reps/*Set 4:* 15 reps |
| | p. 82 | Pull-Up: Close Grip | *Set 1:* 20 reps/*Set 2:* 15 reps/*Set 3:* 10 reps |
| | p. 83 | Pull-Up: Behind the Neck | *Set 1:* 15 reps/*Set 2:* 10 reps/*Set 3:* 5 reps |
| | p. 84 | Dip | 4 x 25 reps |
| | p. 85 | Push-Up: Regular | *Set 1:* 100 reps/*Set 2:* 75 reps/*Set 3:* 50 reps/*Set 4:* 25 reps |
| | p. 86 | Push-Up: Diamond | *Set 1:* 25 reps/*Set 2:* 20 reps/*Set 3:* 15 reps/*Set 4:* 10 reps |
| | p. 92 | Eight-Count Body Builders | 4 x 15 reps |
| | p. 94 | Walking Lunge | 4 x 50 yards |
| CARDIO | | • Monday 3-mile run<br>• Wednesday 1-mile swim (freestyle)<br>• Friday 1-mile interval sprints (sprint on straightaway and jog the corners) | |

NAVY SEAL

# NAVY SEAL

| | p. 104 | Hand to Toes | 1 x 65 reps |
|---|---|---|---|
| | p. 105 | X Sit-Up | 1 x 65 reps |
| | p. 106 | Ranger Crunch | 1 x 65 reps |
| | p. 108 | Hibberty Jibberty | 1 x 65 reps |
| | p. 110 | Obliques | 1 x 65 reps |
| | p. 113 | Lower Ab Crunch | 1 x 65 reps |
| | p. 111 | Flutter Kick | 1 x 45 reps (4 count) |

NAVY SEAL

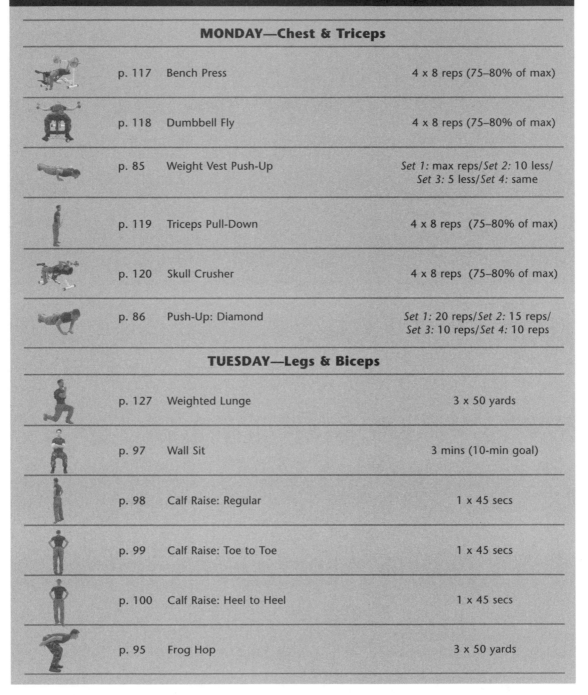

# ALTERNATIVE WORKOUT: WEIGHT-TRAINING PROGRAM

### MONDAY—Chest & Triceps

| | | | |
|---|---|---|---|
| | p. 117 | Bench Press | 4 x 8 reps (75–80% of max) |
| | p. 118 | Dumbbell Fly | 4 x 8 reps (75–80% of max) |
| | p. 85 | Weight Vest Push-Up | *Set 1:* max reps/*Set 2:* 10 less/ *Set 3:* 5 less/*Set 4:* same |
| | p. 119 | Triceps Pull-Down | 4 x 8 reps (75–80% of max) |
| | p. 120 | Skull Crusher | 4 x 8 reps (75–80% of max) |
| | p. 86 | Push-Up: Diamond | *Set 1:* 20 reps/*Set 2:* 15 reps/ *Set 3:* 10 reps/*Set 4:* 10 reps |

### TUESDAY—Legs & Biceps

| | | | |
|---|---|---|---|
| | p. 127 | Weighted Lunge | 3 x 50 yards |
| | p. 97 | Wall Sit | 3 mins (10-min goal) |
| | p. 98 | Calf Raise: Regular | 1 x 45 secs |
| | p. 99 | Calf Raise: Toe to Toe | 1 x 45 secs |
| | p. 100 | Calf Raise: Heel to Heel | 1 x 45 secs |
| | p. 95 | Frog Hop | 3 x 50 yards |

# ALTERNATIVE WORKOUT: WEIGHT-TRAINING PROGRAM

| | | |
|---|---|---|
| p. 128 | Preacher Curl | 4 x 8 reps (75–80% of max) |
| p. 129 | Seated Dumbbell Curl | 4 x 8 reps (75–80% of max) |
| p. 130 | Curl Bar—Inner Grip | 4 x 8 reps (75–80% of max) |

## WEDNESDAY–Shoulders & Back

| | | |
|---|---|---|
| p. 80 | Pull-Up: Regular | 8-10-12-14-12-10-8 |
| p. 82 | Pull-Up: Close Grip | 6-8-10-8-6 |
| p. 83 | Pull-Up: Behind the Neck | 2-4-6-4-2 |
| p. 122 | Lat Pull-Down | 3 x 8 reps (75–80% of max) |
| p. 123 | Military Press | 3 x 8 reps (75–80% of max) |
| p. 125 | Shoulder Raise | 3 x 8 reps (75–80% of max) |
| p. 124 | Shoulder Rotation | 3 x 8 reps (75–80% of max) |

## THURSDAY—Chest & Triceps

| | | |
|---|---|---|
| p. 117 | Bench Press (Super Sets) | *Set 1:* 80% of max/*Set 2:* take off 20 lbs/ *Set 3:* take off 20 lbs/*Set 4:* take off 20 lbs (no rest between sets) |
| p. 118 | Dumbbell Fly (Super Sets) | *Set 1:* 80% of max/*Set 2:* take off 20 lbs/ *Set 3:* take off 20 lbs/*Set 4:* take off 20 lbs (no rest between sets) |
| p. 85 | Weight Vest Push-Up (Super Sets) | *Set 1:* max reps in full vest/*Set 2–n:* take 1 weight out of front & back each set and perform max reps until vest is empty |

# ALTERNATIVE WORKOUT: WEIGHT-TRAINING PROGRAM

| | p. 84 | Dip | 4 x 15–20 reps |
|---|---|---|---|
| | p. 120 | Skull Crusher (Super Sets) | 4 x 8–10 reps |
| | p. 121 | Triceps Kickback | 4 x 8 reps |
| | p. 119 | Triceps Pull-Downs | 4 x 8–10 reps |
| | p. 86 | Push-Up: Diamond | 1 x to failure |

## FRIDAY—Legs & Biceps

| | p. 127 | Weighted Lunge | 3 x 50 yards |
|---|---|---|---|
| | p. 97 | Wall Sit | 3 mins (10-min goal) |
| | p. 98 | Calf Raise: Regular | 1 x 45 secs |
| | p. 99 | Calf Raise: Toe to Toe | 1 x 45 secs |
| | p. 100 | Calf Raise: Heel to Heel | 1 x 45 secs |
| | p. 95 | Frog Hop | 3 x 50 yards |
| | p. 128 | Preacher Curl | 4 x 8 reps (75–80% of max) |
| | p. 129 | Seated Dumbbell Curl | 4 x 8 reps (75–80% of max) |
| | p. 130 | Curl Bar—Inner Grip | 4 x 8 reps (75–80% of max) |

# GOAL & MEASUREMENT CHARTS

**Every 30 Days**      Date _____

Neck _____      Shoulders _____      Chest _____

Waist _____      Thigh _____      Calves _____

Weight (Goal)_____ Weight (Current) _____ Body Fat %_____ Body Fat (Current) _____

**Exercise Calisthenics Max**

Pull-Ups (Goal) _____      Pull-Ups _____      Sit-Ups (Goal) _____      Sit-Ups _____

Push-Ups (Goal) _____      Push-Ups _____      Lunges (Goal) _____      Lunges _____

Dips (Goal) _____      Dips _____

**Free-Weight Exercise Max**

Bench (Goal)_____      Bench _____      Curl (Goal) _____      Curl _____

Squat (Goal)_____      Squat_____      Military Press (Goal) _____      Military Press _____

**Every 30 Days**      Date _____

Neck _____      Shoulders _____      Chest _____

Waist _____      Thigh _____      Calves _____

Weight (Goal) _____ Weight (Current) _____ Body Fat % _____ Body Fat (Current) _____

**Exercise Calisthenics Max**

Pull-Ups (Goal) _____      Pull-Ups _____      Sit-Ups (Goal) _____      Sit-Ups _____

Push-Ups (Goal) _____      Push-Ups _____      Lunges (Goal) _____      Lunges _____

Dips (Goal) _____      Dips _____

**Free-Weight Exercise Max**

Bench (Goal)_____      Bench _____      Curl (Goal) _____      Curl _____

Squat (Goal)_____      Squat_____      Military Press (Goal) _____      Military Press _____

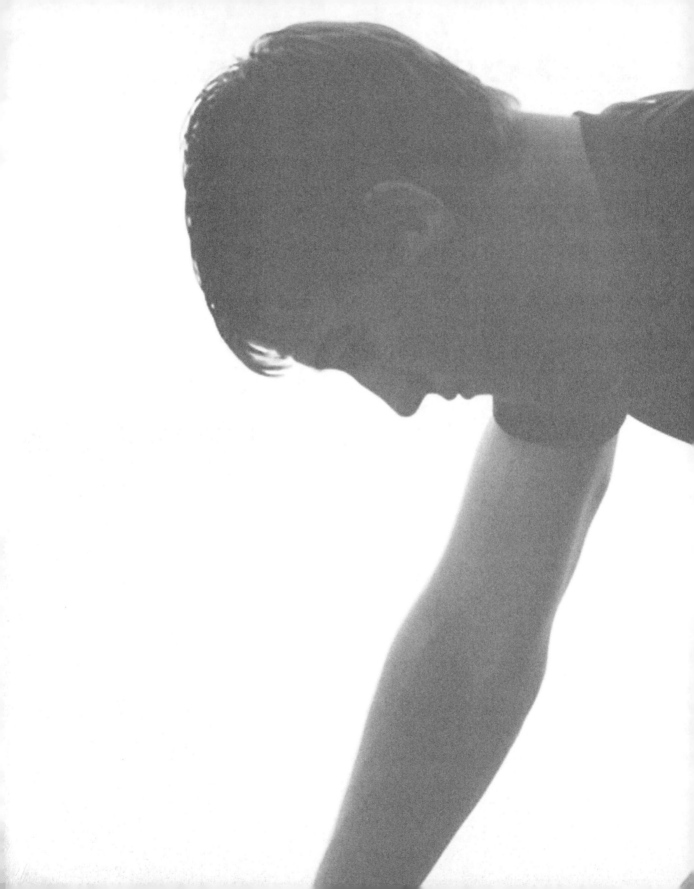

# part 3:

# the

# exercises

# jumping jacks

There's nothing fancy about Jumping Jacks. They're a great vehicle to get the blood pumping through our muscle groups without dramatic strain to the muscle fibers. All Special Operation branches utilize this warm-up.

**STARTING POSITION:** Stand with your feet together, keeping a slight bend in your knees. Place your hands by your sides and look straight ahead.

starting position

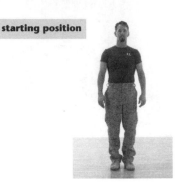

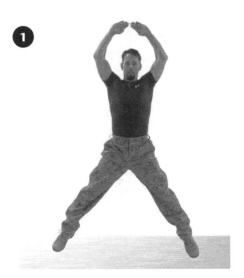

**1** With a light thrust upward, open your feet past the width of your shoulders. At the same time, raise your hands and touch them lightly above your head. Do not cheat yourself by not touching your hands.

**2** Return to starting position, making sure not to slap yourself when your hands return to your hips.

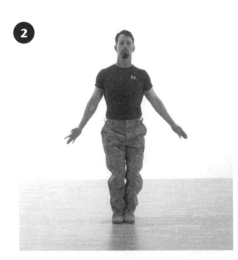

**TIP**

You do not have to jump very high to perform a perfect jumping jack.

# half jumping jacks

*Half Jumping Jacks are a quicker-paced modification of Jumping Jacks to help get the blood flowing. The main differences are that your arms do not go above your shoulders and your pace is two to three times the regular speed. Keep in mind that if you pick up the pace you still must maintain good technique.*

**STARTING POSITION:** Stand with your feet together, keeping a slight bend in your knees. Place your hands by your sides and look straight ahead.

**starting position**

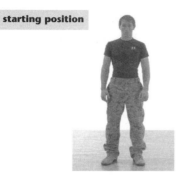

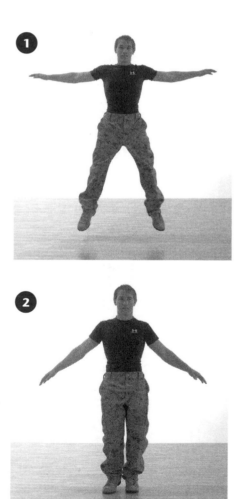

**1** With a light spring, open your feet a little past shoulder width while raising your arms to shoulder height.

**2** Immediately bring your arms and legs back together to starting position.

# iron mikes

*Iron Mikes are identical to lunges and are utilized by the Army Rangers as a warm-up. Although I prefer lower-impact exercises for warm-ups, Iron Mikes are a great leg exercise. Iron Mikes are a four-count exercise (e.g., 1-2-3-1, 1-2-3-2), and I highly recommend taking this exercise slow to make sure that when you step out, you don't let your knees go past the front of your toes.*

**STARTING POSITION:** Stand with your feet parallel and place your hands on your hips. Look straight ahead.

**starting position**

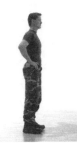

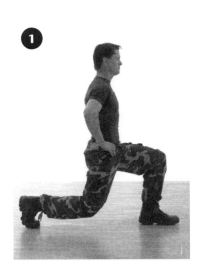

**1** Step straight forward with your left foot, trying not to come down too hard or too fast. Maintain a straight back and keep looking straight ahead. Do not take too large or too short of a step: If you take too short of a step, your knee will go past your toes; if you take too long of a step, you put added stress on your legs for a warm-up.

**2** Return to starting position and step forward with your right leg. Remember to step forward and not back.

**TIP**
Try not to look down at your feet as this will cause your shoulders to lean forward. I recommend practicing in front of a mirror to watch your form.

## chest stretch

*Special Operations relies a lot on the chest. If you don't stretch out your chest, you could end up pulling a muscle, which can affect your entire upper-body routine. Keep in mind that your chest can tighten up during any exercise routine so restretch as you feel necessary.*

**STARTING POSITION:** Stand with your left side to a sturdy, tall object (wall, doorframe), about one foot away, and place your left hand on the object so that it's behind your shoulder and one to two feet above. Make sure your arm is locked straight.

**starting position**

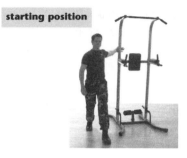

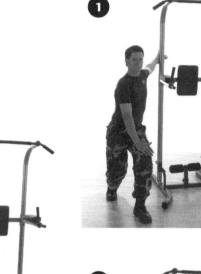

**1** Step your left foot 1–2 feet forward.

**2** Bend your left knee and drop down while pressing forward until you feel the stretch in your chest.

**3** Gently release and switch sides.

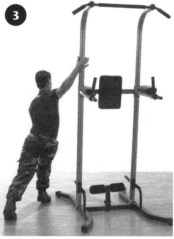

> **TIP**
> Experiment by dropping more forward or downward to get the best stretch. At the same time, you can also adjust your hand position up or down.

## upper back stretch

**STARTING POSITION:** Stand with your feet about hip-width apart. Interlock your fingers in front of you with your palms facing in.

starting position

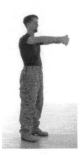

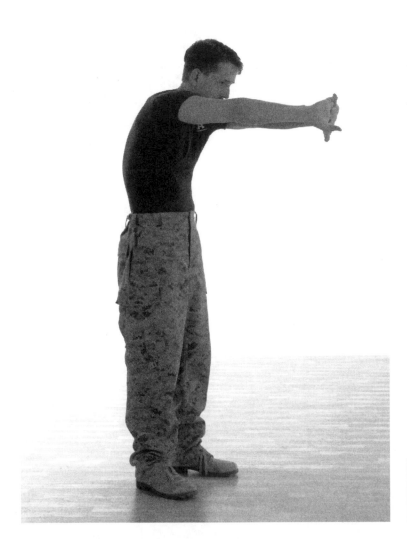

**1** Facing your palms outward, drive your hands forward until your arms are locked straight. Hold and maintain this position for at least 10 seconds. As you finish this stretch, take a deep breath and let your shoulders roll forward. This will allow you to further relax and get the most out of this stretch.

**TIP**
For better balance, you can widen your stance.

# forearm stretch

*You will be surprised how much your forearm can tighten up during exercise, especially during pull-ups. This is a simple stretch but well worth it.*

**STARTING POSITION:** Stand with your feet shoulder-width apart.

**starting position**

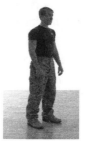

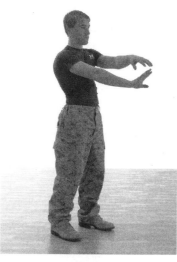

**1** Extend your right hand in front of you and point your fingers straight up. Keep your arm as straight as possible.

**2** Grasp your right fingers with your left hand and slowly pull your fingers and hand towards you.

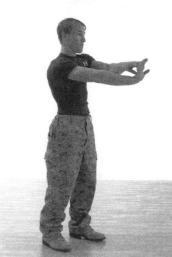

# triceps stretch

*Triceps are essential in your upper body workouts so take the time to stretch them out to prevent injury. Do not rush this stretch, which not only hits your triceps but also the entire side of your back and core; you need to completely relax your back and shoulders while stretching your triceps.*

**STARTING POSITION:** Stand with your feet wider than shoulder-width apart. Adjust the width of your stance to get the most out of this stretch

starting position

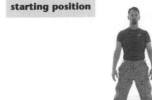

**1** Reach your right hand over your head and touch your upper spine. Place your left hand on your right elbow.

**2** Slowly lean to your left, continuously applying pressure to your right elbow. Go to the point of discomfort but not pain; do not twist your upper body.

**3** Slowly return to starting position and switch sides.

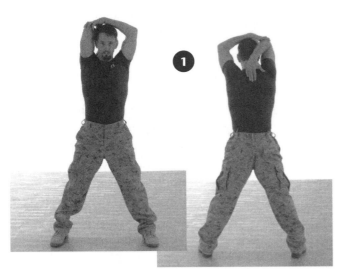

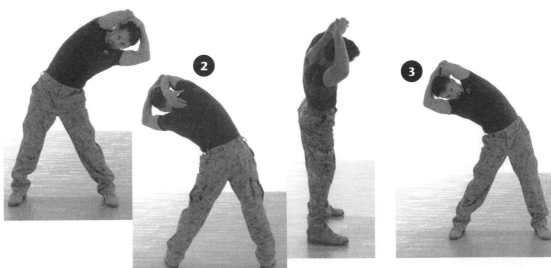

# partner-assisted upper body stretch

*With the assistance of a partner, you can stretch out your upper and lower back while your partner stretches his core, chest, and shoulders at the same time. It is important to take your time on this stretch and lift each other slowly. Pay attention to each other's commands.*

**STARTING POSITION:** Stand back to back and interlock your arms at the elbows. Keep your feet shoulder-width apart for balance.

**starting position**

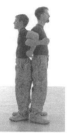

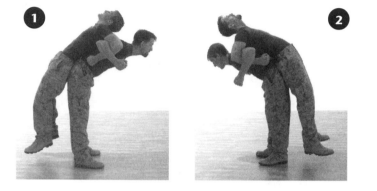

**1** Slowly bend forward to lift your partner's feet just a foot or two off the ground. Don't bend too far forward, which will cause your partner's weight to ride high on your upper body.

**2** Return to starting position and switch roles.

> **TIP**
> Instead of just interlocking your arms, you can also grab your hands to secure this position even better.

# partner-assisted chest stretch     *chest, shoulders*

*This is a great stretch but requires slow movements and relaxation.*

**STARTING POSITION:** *Stand with your feet wider than hip-width apart and raise your arms until they're about shoulder height. Your partner stands behind you with one leg forward and one leg back for balance. He then grabs both of your wrists from underneath for more control.*

**starting position**

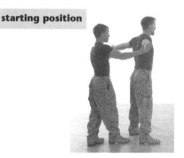

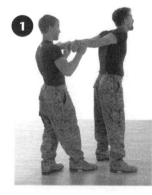

**1** Your partner slowly pulls your arms backward while maintaining them at shoulder height. Tell your partner when you get close to your peak—go to the point of discomfort but not to the point of pain.

Return to starting position and switch roles.

# side-to-side stretch

**STARTING POSITION:** Stand with your feet wider than shoulder-width apart.

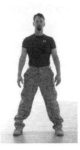

**1** Place your left hand on your left hip and reach your right hand over your head. Keep your right arm a foot or two above your head with a slight bend in your elbow.

**2** Lean to your left while maintaining your right hand above your head; keep driving with this arm. Do not rotate your hip during this movement.

**3** Return to starting position and switch sides.

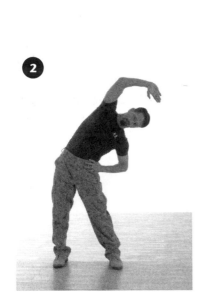

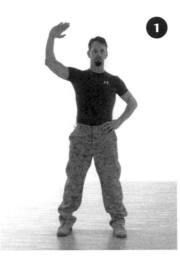

# v stretch

**STARTING POSITION:** Sit on the floor with your legs extended in front of you and your feet a foot or two wider than shoulder width. Sit up tall, bending your knees slightly if necessary to release any tension in your back and knees.

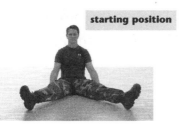

starting position

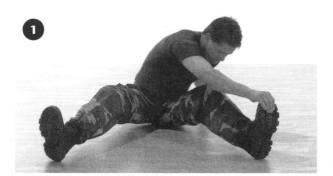

**1** Grab your left foot with your right hand and place your left hand on the ground behind your left hip. Push with your left hand to help you get more out of the stretch.

**2** Take a deep breath as you slowly bring your chest and head towards your left knee.

**3** Slowly return to starting position and switch sides.

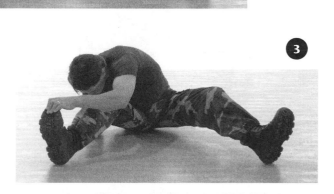

## straight-leg stretch

*Straight-leg stretches are a great transition from V stretches (page 65).*

**STARTING POSITION:** Sit on the floor with your legs together and extended in front of you. Bend your knees slightly.

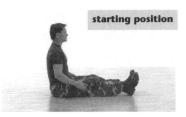

starting position

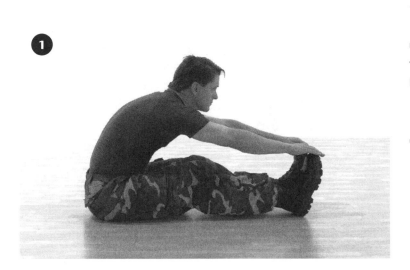

**1**

**1** Grab your toes with your fingers and relax your entire upper body. This will allow you to stretch your hamstrings better.

**2** Bring your chest and head toward your knees.

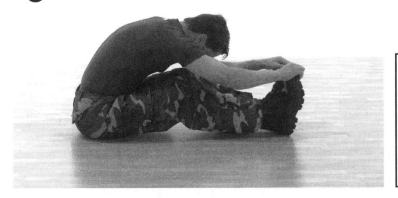

**2**

**TIP**

As you become more flexible, walk your fingers down the bottom of your shoes or place your hands over the tops of your feet. Eventually your fingertips will hit the floor near the base of your heels.

# ITB stretch

*If you have a tight lower back, you need to stretch more than just your lower back muscles. Even though the iliotibial band (ITB) is a good place to start, you'll still need to target your hamstrings and calves. This version allows you to get more leverage.*

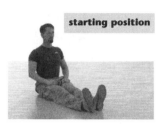

starting position

**STARTING POSITION:** Sit on the floor with your legs straight out in front of you.

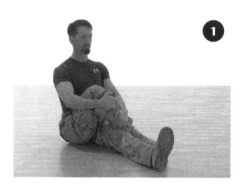

**1** Place your right foot on the outside of your left knee. Wrap your arms around your right knee; you can also grab your right elbow with your left hand for leverage. Apply pressure by squeezing your leg to your chest. Don't be afraid to put a good squeeze on your leg. The glute muscle is very resilient and needs a lot of pressure to loosen up.

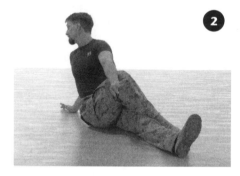

**2** Slowly release and place your left arm on the outside of your right knee while locking your arm straight. Place your right arm behind your right hip. Now look over your right shoulder as you apply pressure to your right leg with your left arm. Rotate your right shoulder to the right until you feel tension in the lower back. Hold this position until the tension releases. Take a deep breath to get your lower back to stretch a little more.

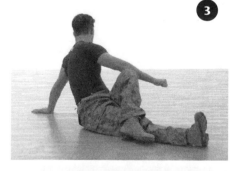

**3** Return to starting position and switch sides.

### MODIFICATION FOR TENDER KNEE
Place your left hand on your right ankle and place your right hand on your left knee. Squeeze with even pressure while lifting the right foot off the ground.

# hamstring stretch

*Rangers utilize a three-part hamstring stretch and top it off by stretching the calves. Your hand position helps you maintain control.*

**STARTING POSITION:** Sit on the floor with your legs straight out in front of you, keeping a slight bend in your knees. Place one hand beneath each leg. Take a deep breath and relax your entire upper body and legs. Slowly lower your chin down towards your thighs.

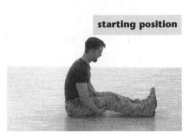

starting position

**1** Keeping your current body position as much as you can, move your hands until they're beneath your knees, then lower your body once more. Do not look down at your belly button—stare straight ahead as you lower your chin.

**1**

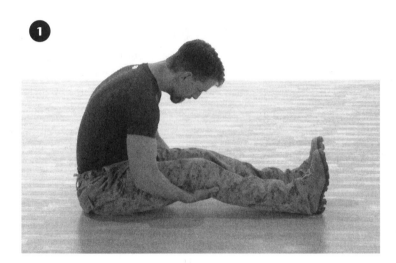

**2** Release the pressure slightly and move your hands until they're beneath your lower calves. Lower your head towards your knees and let your gaze fall to your knees. If possible, grab your toes and pull them towards you.

**2**

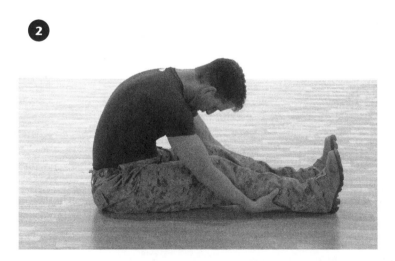

## trunk stretch

*Proper breathing will definitely enhance your stretch. So remember to take a deep breath and let it out slowly after you have reached the peak of your stretch. This will allow you to go a little further.*

**STARTING POSITION:** Lie on your back with your legs extended along the floor and your arms by your sides.

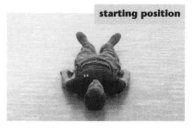
**starting position**

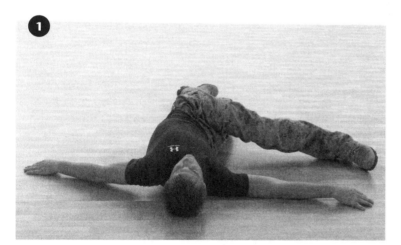

**1** Cross your left leg to your right side, extending your arms into a "T" position. Keep both shoulders on the ground.

Once you have reached and maintained your peak position during the stretch, switch sides.

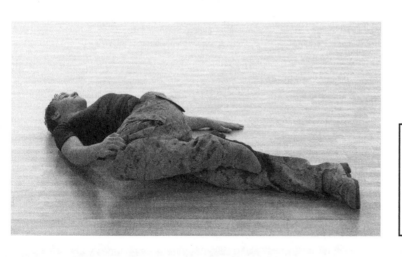

**MODIFICATION**
This can also be done with a bent leg by placing your left foot on the inside of your right knee and then pulling your left knee to your right by using your right hand.

## groin stretch

*There is nothing worse than a pulled groin so take advantage of this stretch and do it as often as you can. The key to groin stretches is taking your time dropping into position and raising up and out of the down position.*

**STARTING POSITION:** Stand with your feet one to two feet wider than shoulder width. Make sure both feet are pointing straight ahead.

**starting position**

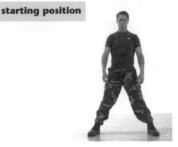

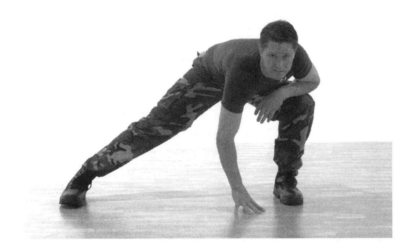

**1** Bend your left knee and place your left elbow on that knee; lean to your left. Once you reach the point where your right foot wants to lift off the ground, lower your hips until you feel discomfort but not pain. Keep your back straight and look forward.

**2** Slowly return to starting position and switch sides.

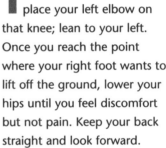

**TIPS**
• Do not sit down too much—it is not necessary to sit all the way down on your heel.
• Keep both feet flat on the ground.

## partner-assisted butterfly stretch

**STARTING POSITION:** Sit with the bottoms of your feet pressed together with your hands on your shoelaces.

starting position

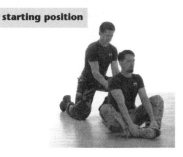

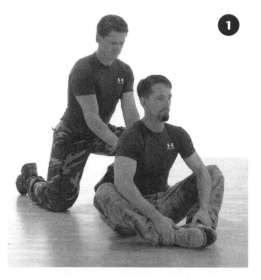

**1** Press your elbows into your inner knees.

**2** From behind, your partner begins to slowly, lightly push forward and down on your lower shoulder blades.

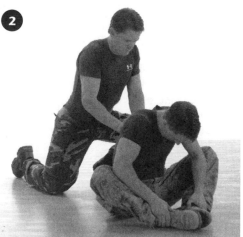

# quad stretch

**STARTING POSITION:** Stand with your feet shoulder-width apart.

starting position

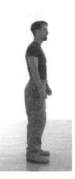

**1** Grab your left foot with your right hand. Keep your back straight and look straight ahead.

**2** Slowly raise your left foot up towards your lower middle back. Take a deep breath, let it out slowly, then apply a little more pressure.

Slowly return to starting position and switch sides.

**TIP**
Keep your abs tight to maintain a straight torso while you stretch.

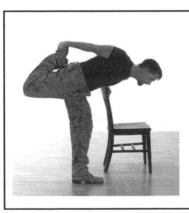

**VARIATION**
For an additional stretch, once you begin to feel pressure as you're raising your foot, slowly bend over and try to lift your knee higher than your hip. You can use a chair for support.

# calf stretch #1

**STARTING POSITION:** Place your hands on the floor as if you were going to perform a push-up.

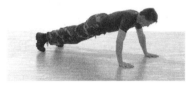
starting position

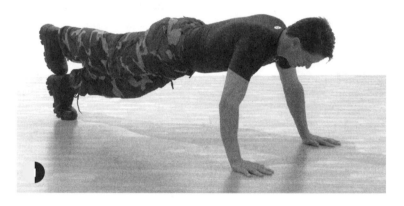

**1** Place the tip of your right foot on top of your left heel.

**2** Lower your left heel to the ground by pushing with your legs and walking your hands towards your feet. Try not to raise your butt too high in the air because this will take away from the stretch.

Return to starting position and switch sides.

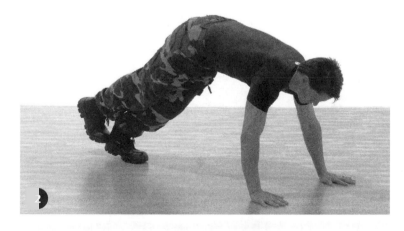

**TIP**

If you can touch your heel to the ground but still don't feel the stretch, bend your elbows and lower your chest towards the ground.

# calf stretch #2

*The key to this stretch is maintaining good balance. Do not place your right and left foot on a single line—allow some distance between the two (width not length).*

**STARTING POSITION:** Stand with your feet shoulder-width apart.

**starting position**

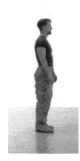

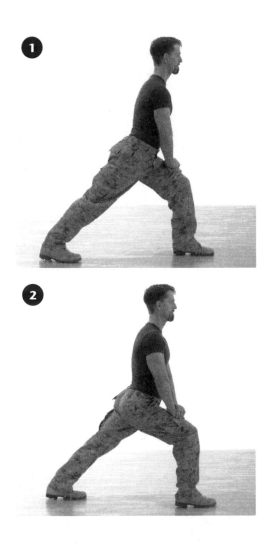

**1** Step your left leg forward and bend your left thigh 90 degrees; place both hands on your left thigh. Extend your right leg further behind you so that your heel is elevated. You should feel tightness in your calf at this point. Lower your heel until it is flat on the ground. As you do so, bring your hips forward and lower them slightly, keeping your back straight.

**2** Switch sides.

**TIPS**
• Use your forward leg for support but do not put all your balance forward on the leg.
• Try to keep your weight centered over your hips.

## cobra stretch

*I like to perform this stretch after every three ab exercises.*

**STARTING POSITION:** Lie flat on your front with your hips firmly down and your hands on the floor, slightly wider than your shoulders. Your feet can be together or shoulder-width apart.

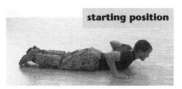
starting position

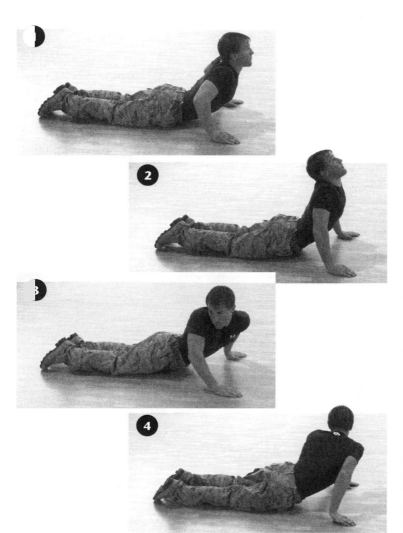

**1–2** Slowly raise your upper body by straightening your arms, exhaling at the point of discomfort. Once you have fully extended your arms, you can tilt your head backwards. Begin to shrug your shoulders towards your ears.

**3** Lower down halfway and drive your left shoulder to the right. Look over your right shoulder until you see your left foot. Hold this position for a few seconds.

**4** Return to center and switch sides.

**TIP**
Perform the Cat Back Stretch (page 76) after this stretch to really stretch out your core.

## cat back stretch

*Always perform this stretch right after the Cobra Stretch.*

**STARTING POSITION:** Come to all fours, placing your hands on the floor and your knees shoulder-width apart.

**starting position**

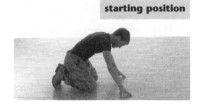

**1** Round your back towards the ceiling like a cat, walking your hands slightly inward toward your knees to raise your lower back.

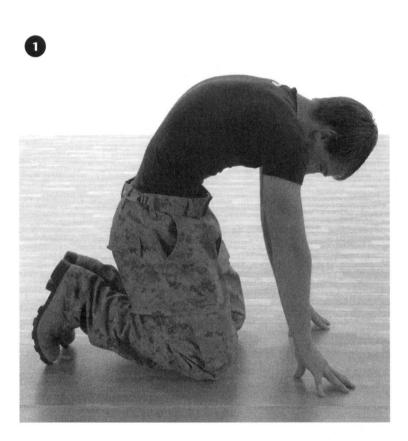

## partner-assisted lower back twist

**STARTING POSITION:** Lie on your back with both legs straight along the floor.

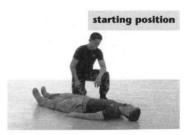
starting position

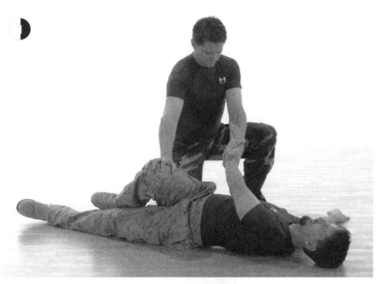

**1** Place your right foot on the inside of your left knee. Your partner kneels down behind your right knee and places his right hand on your right knee. At the same time, he grabs your left arm by the wrist while you grab his arm by his wrist.

**2** He slowly pulls on your left arm while applying pressure to your right knee. Let him know if he needs to apply more pressure or back off.

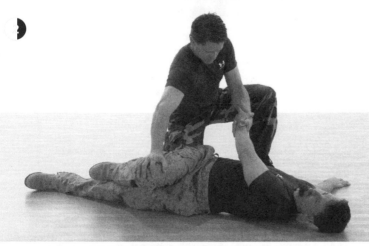

# partner-assisted lower back stretch

*This is one of the best stretches to alleviate lower back pain. Your partner must watch your facial expression to determine that he is taking you to the point of discomfort but not pain.*

**STARTING POSITION:** Lie on your back with both legs straight along the floor. Your partner kneels on your right side and raises your right leg by placing one hand behind your right heel and his other hand on top of your right knee. The key is to elevate your leg without bending it.

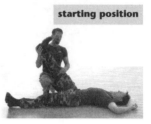

starting position

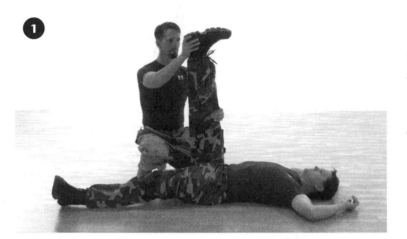

**1** Your partner lifts your leg to the point of discomfort. Hold this position for 3 to 5 seconds.

**2** He lowers it down by one foot to relieve the tension. Hold for 3 to 5 seconds.

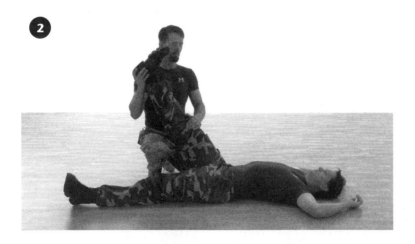

**3** As he lifts the leg again, inhale deeply and exhale slowly at the point of discomfort. As you exhale, your partner applies just a little more pressure. Repeat three times total.

**4** Once he has stretched out your hamstrings and lower back three times, he will lower your leg just six inches. Keeping one hand behind your heel, he places the other hand over the tips of your toes. Maintaining the heel securely, he applies pressure to your toes to stretch your calf.

Switch legs; partner will move to the other side.

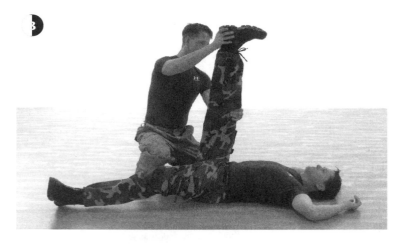

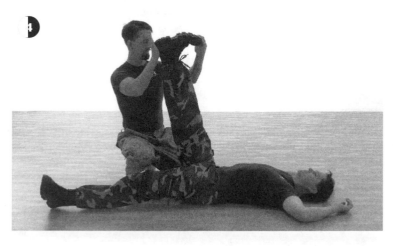

**VARIATION**

This can also be done without a partner by looping a strap or towel around your foot.

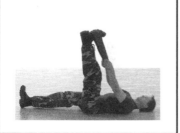

# pull-up—regular

*Special Ops Spin: Pull-ups are so important that every branch of Special Forces incorporates them into their routines. Navy SEALs must be able to lift themselves up onto enemy ships for ship attacks. When fast-roping out of a helicopter, Force Recon and Green Berets must have the upper body strength to slow down their descent. Army Rangers and PJs must scales walls to rescue hostages or downed pilots.*

**STARTING POSITION:** Place your hands on the bar six inches wider than your shoulders; either tuck your thumbs underneath or wrap them around the bar. Drive your elbows down while keeping your chest forward. Cross your ankles and bend your knees 90 degrees.

**starting position**

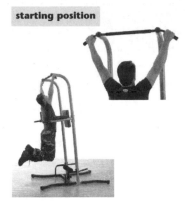

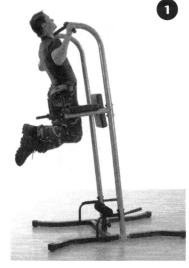

**1** Raise your chin to bar level, keeping your abs tight to help maintain a straight back.

**2** Lower down slowly to starting position.

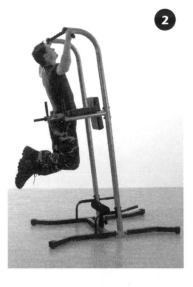

**TIPS**

• If you look in a mirror and see that your arms and hands form a good V, you're in the right position.

• Bending your knees and crossing your ankles keep you from losing proper form while performing a perfect pull-up.

• Do not come down too fast— swinging puts extra pressure on your shoulder joints.

• Make sure not to cheat yourself of excellent back development by doing half pull-ups.

## VARIATION—PARTNER ASSIST

Your partner places his left hand beneath your ankle or right on your shoelaces. His right hand grabs the tip of the shoe so that his palm rests against the sole of the shoe. He now lays his forearm and elbow against his right thigh, allowing the leg to bear the brunt of the pressure. You will push into him when you perform the pull-ups—if he has proper form, this will not be a strain for him.

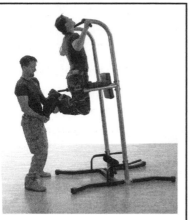

## VARIATION—CHAIR ASSIST

The most difficult part about chair assist is trying not to rely too much on your legs. If your arms are not shaking by your second-to-last rep, you are using your legs too much.

#1 Cross your ankles and place the ball of your lower foot on the chair. To perform the pull-up, use your thigh muscles to drive your body upward while contracting your back muscles.

#2 Place your feet together on the chair and drive off the ball of your feet, using your thigh muscles to assist in the pull-up. Keep your abs tight to prevent your back from bowing.

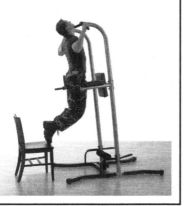

## pull-up—close grip

*Special Ops Spin: Special Ops operators use the shoulder blades, fore-arms, and triceps in a number of scenarios, including cast and recovery, enemy takedowns, and crawling along the jungle floor.*

**STARTING POSITION:** Place your hands on the bar one to two inches apart; either tuck your thumbs underneath or wrap them around the bar. Bring your elbows in tight and maintain this position throughout the movement.

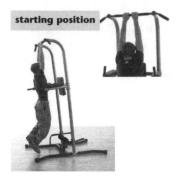

starting position

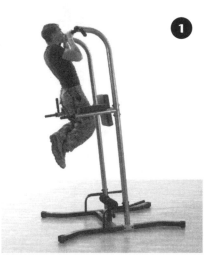

**1** Raise your chin to bar level, keeping your abs tight to help maintain a straight back.

**2** Slowly lower down to starting position.

# pull-up—behind the neck

*Special Ops Spin: The inner back and shoulder blade muscles play a key role in any climbing or elevating movement, which is a common activity in Special Operations.*

*This is also one of the toughest pull-up exercises you'll ever do.*

**STARTING POSITION:** Place your hands on the bar so that they're slightly wider than your regular pull-up grip; either tuck your thumbs underneath or wrap them around the bar. Cross your ankles and bend your knees 90 degrees.

**starting position**

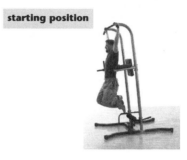

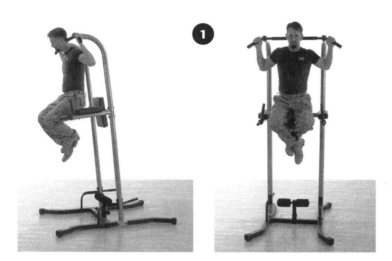

**1** With your head tilted slightly forward, raise yourself up until the base of your skull is at bar level. Aim for your hair line and keep your abs tight to help maintain a straight back

**2** Slowly lower down to starting position.

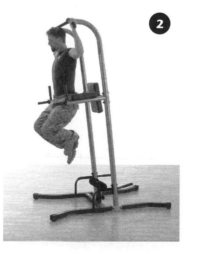

**TIP**
Maintain a smooth, fluid motion throughout the entire movement, both up and down.

## dip

*Special Ops Spin: During shipboard attacks, the dip movement is a key element when it comes to transitioning from climbing the side of a ship to boarding it. Any movement that would require a soldier to climb a wall or obstacle incorporates similar muscular exertion.*

*When doing dips, the height from which you drop down is really important. Most people either do not drop low enough or drop too low. The former will not allow you to get the most out of this exercise, and the latter puts too much strain on the shoulders.*

starting position

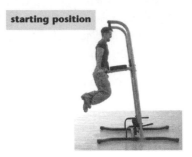

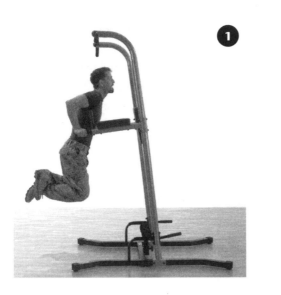

**①**

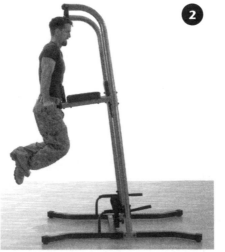

**②**

**STARTING POSITION:** Place your hands on the bars so that your hands are directly under your shoulders. Keep your shoulders away from your ears. Cross your ankles and keep your abs tight throughout the movement to help keep you from swinging. Look straight ahead and maintain a straight back.

**1** Lower yourself at a controlled pace, stopping when your elbows are bent 90 degrees.

**2** Apply pressure with your triceps to push yourself back up, stopping once your arms are fully extended.

---

**TIP**
• Look in a mirror while you perform this so you can get an idea of the correct dip height.
• Do not position yourself too far back on the bar.

# push-up—regular

*Special Ops Spin: The military has been utilizing regular push-ups for decades since they're essential for developing the frequently used chest muscles, triceps, and abs. Imagine an operator in the middle of a fire-fight with 80 pounds of gear on his back when someone yells out, "I have an exit!" This operator requires chest and triceps muscles to help him spring to his feet.*

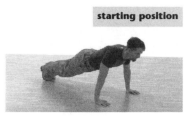
**starting position**

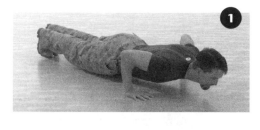

**STARTING POSITION:** Place your hands on the floor so that they're slightly wider than shoulder width. Your elbows should not flare out past your hands. Place your feet side by side or one foot on top of the other. Maintain a straight line from your shoulders to your feet by keeping your abs tight; do not let your back sag or raise your seat too high in the air. Imagine you have a 2 x 4 down your back.

**1** Lower down until your chest is one or two inches from the ground.

**2** Press up to starting position.

---

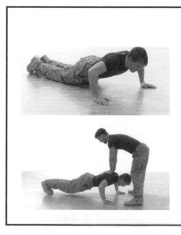

### VARIATION

If you have trouble doing this from your feet, start from your knees until you develop the strength to get off your knees.

### VARIATION—PARTNER ASSIST

Keep your abs very tight during this one. Your partner stands in front of you and places one hand on each shoulder blade. As you drop down to the halfway mark, your partner applies medium pressure on your shoulders. Your partner must maintain a consistent level of pressure throughout the exercise; he may even have to ease off if you start to drop, or else yell encouragement. If you run out of strength and drop down to the ground, don't stop. Get back up and last as long as you can. If you fall during the first 15 of 60 seconds, then it just means that you have to keep getting back up for 45 more seconds.

## push-up—diamond

*Special Ops Spin: Triceps are important in any pushing or pulling movement. Just about every operation will require great strength from this muscle group.*

*The key to getting the most out of Diamond Push-Ups is hand position. If you have your hands too far forward, you'll feel it more in your shoulders.*

**STARTING POSITION:** Place your hands on the ground and touch your fingers and thumbs together. Extend your legs behind you and place your feet a little wider than shoulder-width apart. Keep your abs tight as you bring your hands just under your lower chest.

**starting position**

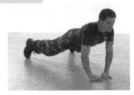

**1** Lower yourself down to within one inch of the ground—come as close as you can to your sternum with your hands. Let your elbows flare out to hit your triceps harder.

**2** Press up to starting position.

**1**

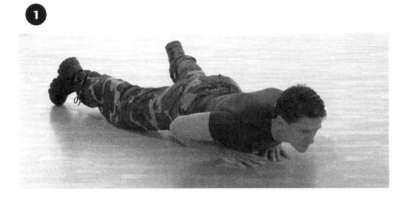

**2**

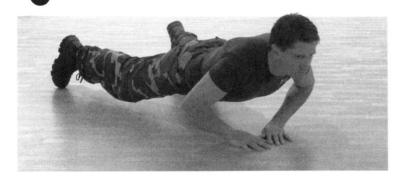

**TIP**
If you get a cramp in your hip, position your feet closer together.

# push-up—ranger diamond

*Special Ops Spin: Just about every Special Ops mission depends on triceps strength. This is a favorite of the Army Rangers.*

*Ranger Diamond Push-Ups differ from normal Diamond Push-Ups in that only your thumbs touch; here, your fingers are extended forward and your hand position looks like a U. In addition, your elbows are tucked in instead of flared out.*

**starting position**

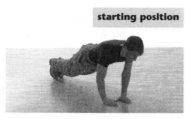

**STARTING POSITION:** Place your hands on the ground and touch your thumbs together, letting your fingers extend forward. Your hands should be under your chest. Extend your legs behind you and place your feet together. Keep your abs tight and your elbows close to your sides throughout the movement.

**1** Lower down until you are one or two inches from the ground, making sure your elbows stay in.

**2** Press up to starting position.

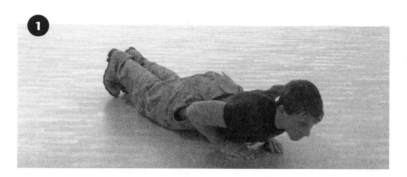

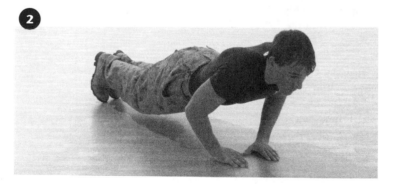

# push-up—triple sets

*This is a combination of wide-angle, regular, and diamond push-ups. You perform each exercise as one rep then move onto the next position. Wide Angle counts as rep 1, Regular as rep 2 and Diamond as rep 3— this completes one cycle or 1-2-3-1, 1-2-3-2, 1-2-3-3, etc.*

**STARTING POSITION:** Place your hands six inches wider than regular push-ups and your legs side by side. Keep your abs tight to maintain a straight back.

starting position

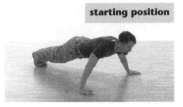

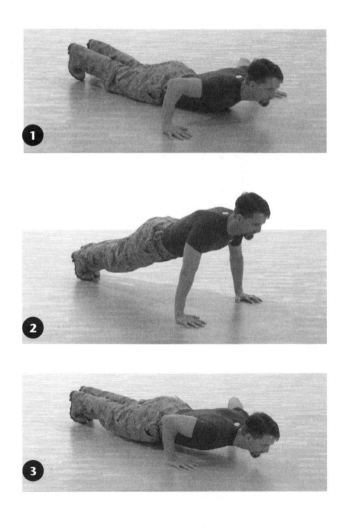

**1** From this wide-angle push-up position, drop down until you're one to two inches from the ground.

**2** Immediately switch to a regular push-up as you press up, making sure hands are directly to the sides of your shoulders.

**3** Lower down until you're one to two inches from the ground.

**4** Immediately switch to a diamond push-up as you press up, touching your fingers and thumbs together and moving your feet a little wider than shoulder-width apart. Your hands should be just under your lower chest.

**5** Lower yourself down to within one inch of the ground, coming as close as you can to your sternum with your hands. Let your elbows flare out.

**6** Press back up to the wide-angle push-up position.

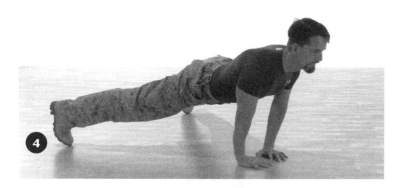

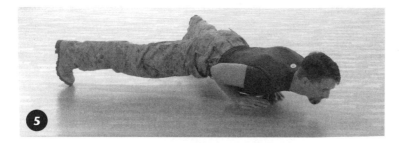

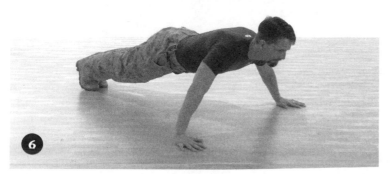

# push-up—elevated

*Special Ops Spin: Just about every Special Ops mission depends on triceps strength.*

*This exercise requires strong abs so if you're just beginning, you might want to hold off on this one until you're stronger. Basically, you perform push-ups from three different positions. A chair or bench is good for the top position, and stairs or a crate can work for the middle position. It is very important to maintain tight abs throughout the entire movement to prevent your back from sagging.*

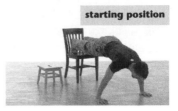

starting position

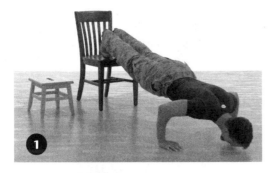

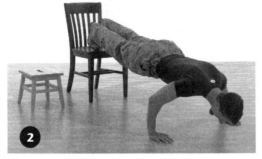

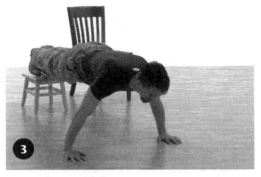

**STARTING POSITION:** Place your hands in a regular push-up position (hands directly to the sides of your shoulders, legs together). Start with your feet at least 3 feet up in the air.

**1** Lower down and touch your nose to the floor.

**2** Press back up and continue with your reps at this level.

**3** Once you've completed your set and taken the prescribed rest, lower your feet until they're 1.5 to 2 feet from the ground.

**4** Lower down and touch your nose to the floor.

**5** Press back up and continue with your reps at this level.

**6** Once you've completed your set, release your feet to the ground so that you're in regular push-up position.

**7** Lower down until you're one inch from the floor.

**8** Press back up and finish your reps.

**TIP**
I recommend performing this exercise in front of a mirror so you can watch your form.

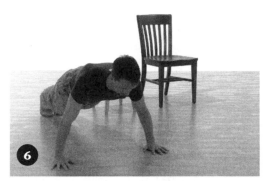

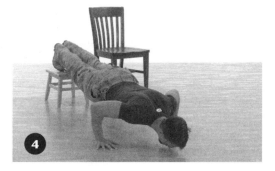

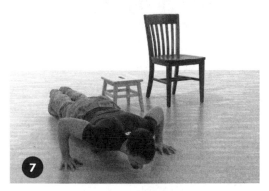

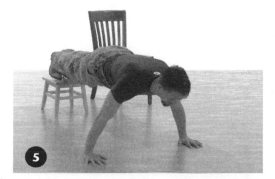

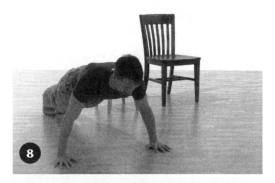

# eight-count body builders

*Special Ops Spin: Eight-Count Body Builders are an excellent way to develop the muscles used when crawling on your belly or engaging in a firefight that requires getting up and down a lot.*

*This is a great way to incorporate cardio, upper body, and lower body and also develop your quick-burst muscle fibers while working on endurance.*

**STARTING POSITION:** Stand with your feet together and place your hands on your hips.

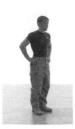

starting position

**1** Squat down and place your hands on the ground.

**2** Thrust your feet back until you're in a push-up position.

**3** Open your feet until they're wider than shoulder-width apart.

**4** Jump your feet back to push-up position.

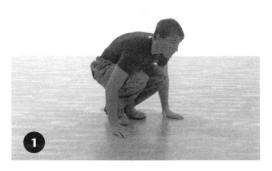

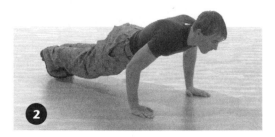

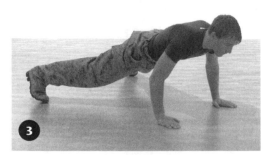

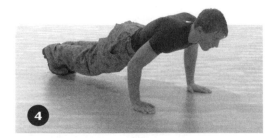

**5**  Lower down for a regular push-up.

**6** Press yourself back up.

**7** Jump your feet back to the squat position.

**8** Return to starting position.

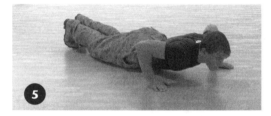

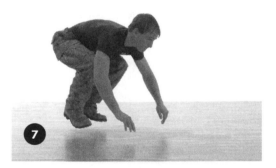

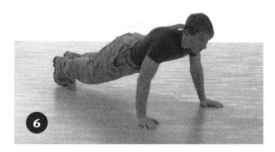

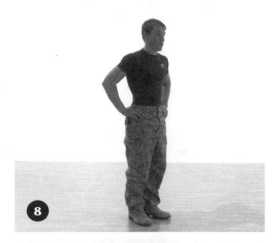

## walking lunge

*Special Ops Spin: Walking Lunges enable any Special Ops platoon to have one leg up on the enemy. Rangers and Green Beret are known for long patrols where leg strength and endurance are essential for completing the mission. Recon could be called upon for missions that require everything from long dives to reconnaissance deep within enemy territory. SEALs may have to swim half a mile onto shore and then take on the enemy. If a downed pilot is injured, PJs literally have to carry him out with the enemy bearing down on them. These lunges are going to help them get there.*

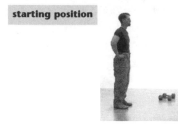

starting position

**STARTING POSITION:** Stand with your feet together and hands on your hips.

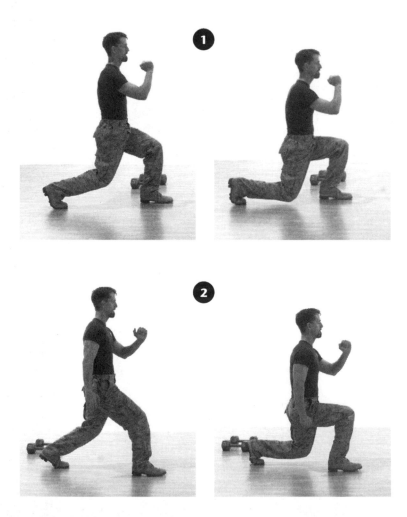

**1** Step your left foot forward into a lunge, making sure that your knee does not cross over the tip of your shoe; keep your back straight and chin up. Bend your right arm up.

**2** Without stopping in the middle or standing up, step your left foot forward into a lunge.

Continue alternating legs.

# frog hop

*Special Ops Spin: When you're in a firefight and your right-hand man finds an exit to the left, you must be able spring to your feet, utilizing every fast-twitch muscle in your lower body, in order to get out of there quickly.*

*Frog Hops are a good exercise to get your lungs burning.*

**STARTING POSITION:** Stand with your legs shoulder-width apart and your arms in front of you like a downhill skier.

**starting position**

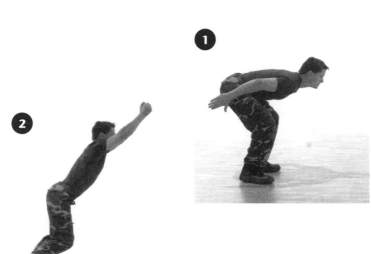

**1** Move your arms back into the exploding position and squat down slightly to coil your legs.

**2** Bring your arms forward and simultaneously explode forward, not up. Be sure to land with your knees soft, not stiff.

**3** Bring your arms back to prepare for the next jump.

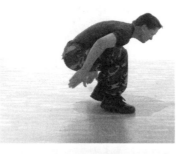

**TIP**
Do not recoil your arms back until after you have landed.

## star hop

*Special Ops Spin: Leg strength and speed is essential after you've eliminated your target. You must get out of there quickly and efficiently, running, hopping over obstacles, and hurdling ditches in an attempt to return to your evac (evacuation) point as fast as you can.*

*Star Hops work the quick-burst/fast-twitch muscles and will increase your vertical leap and lung capacity.*

**starting position**

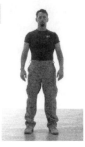

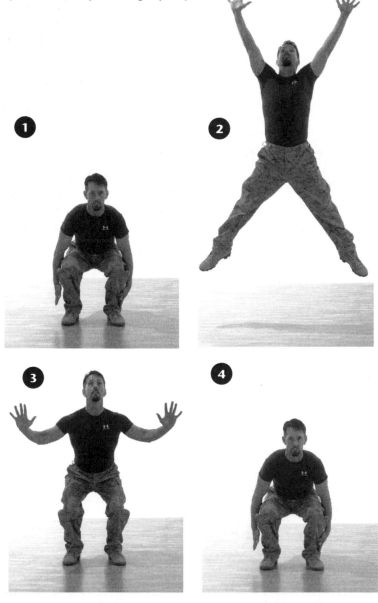

**STARTING POSITION:** Stand with your legs shoulder-width apart.

**1** Squat down so that you can place your hands on the outside of each ankle.

**2** Explode upward as high as you can, reaching up with your hands, which are slightly wider than your shoulders. Keep your back straight, your chin up, and your rear end down.

**3** Land softly with your knees bent to absorb any recoil.

**4** Squat back down and prepare to explode again.

# wall sit

*Special Ops Spin: During an ambush, squatting for hours at a time is a reality that requires much endurance that can be gained through Wall Sits.*

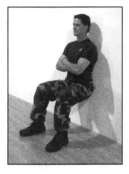

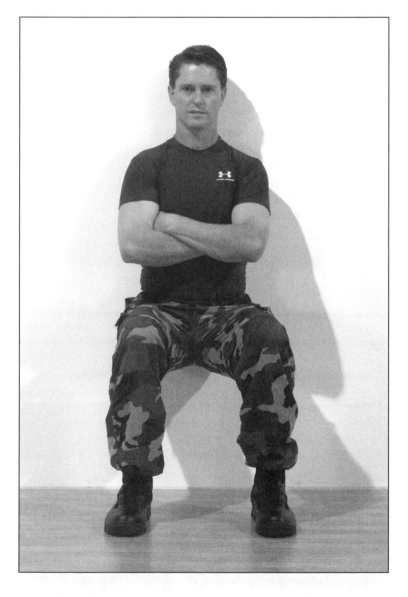

**THE POSITION:** With your back flush against a wall, walk your feet forward until your knees are bent 90 degrees and do not cross over your toes. Your knees should be shoulder-width apart. You can cross your arms across your chest. Hold the position, making sure to keep your back straight and not lean forward.

**TIP**
Do not place your hands on your knees—this is cheating.

# calf raise—regular

*Special Ops Spin: Any type of long march, run, or swim requires strong calves; any weakness in this area can jeopardize your ability to contribute to your squad or platoon.*

*To get the most out of calf raises, you must keep your legs completely straight. If you bend your knees at all, your quads kick in.*

**STARTING POSITION:** Stand with your feet shoulder-width apart and place your hands on your hips.

starting position

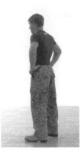

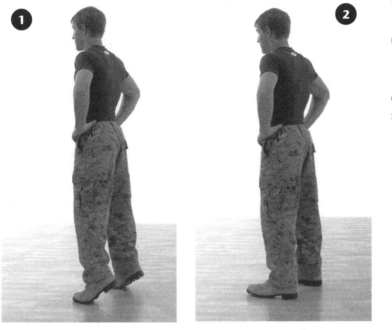

**1** Rise onto the balls of your feet so that your heels are up at least 2 inches.

**2** Lower down with control. Try to maintain the same speed both up and down.

# calf raise—toe to toe

**STARTING POSITION:** Stand with your toes touching each other with your heels flared out; make sure your toes touch throughout the exercise. Hands can be at your sides or on your hips.

starting position

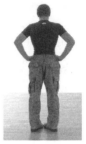

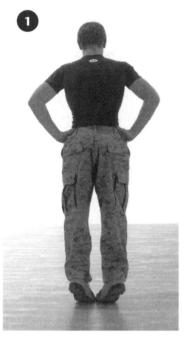

**1** Rise up onto the balls of your feet, making sure your toes keep touching.

**2** Lower down with control. Check that your toes are touching before continuing.

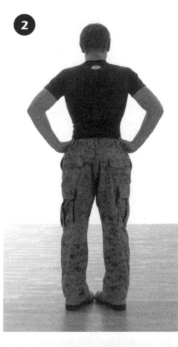

**TIP**
If you have balance issues, you can hold on to a pole or wall until you are able to shift your hands to your hips.

## calf raise—heel to heel

**STARTING POSITION:** Stand with your heels touching each other with your toes pointed outward. Try to keep your legs as straight as possible throughout this movement. Hands can be at your sides or on your hips.

starting position

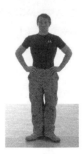

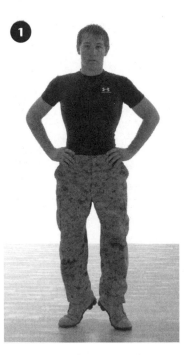

**1** Rise up onto the balls of your feet, making sure your heels keep touching.

**2** Lower down with control. Check that your heels are touching before continuing.

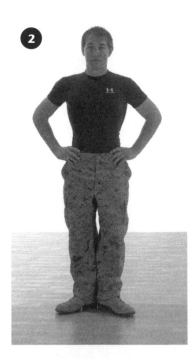

**TIP**
• The degree of difficulty can be increased by reps, time, and weight, or by utilizing a box, step, or other object to increase the range of motion.
• If you have balance issues, you can hold on to a pole, chair, or wall until you are able to shift your hands to your hips.

# bench back exercise

*Special Ops Spin: The lower back definitely comes into play when your buddy goes down and you have to lift him up over your shoulders or over an obstacle. If your lower back is not strong enough, you'll put yourself in jeopardy of hurting yourself and further sacrifice the mission.*

*This exercise can be performed off the ground or a bench. I recommend beginning on the ground and working your way up to the bench.*

**STARTING POSITION:** Lie belly-down on a bench and interlock your fingers behind your head. Your partner grips behind your heels or ankles; he must maintain a solid grip throughout the exercise.

**starting position**

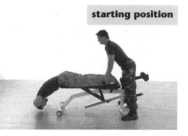

**1** Raise your upper body as high as you feel comfortable by contracting your lower back.

**2** Maintain control as you come back down.

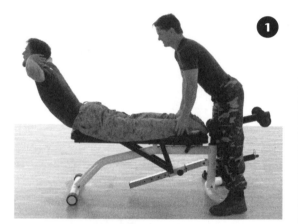

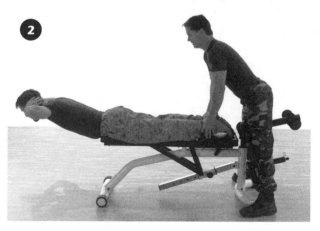

**GROUND VARIATION**
This can also be done on the ground.

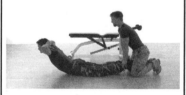

**MODIFICATION**
When performing this on the bench, your partner can also sit on your lower legs.

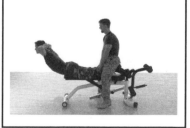

# ruck sack march (with airborne shuffle)

*Special Ops Spin: This is a terrific exercise to help prepare your legs for the rigors of patrolling.*

*Equipment:*

• *A sand bag filled with 30 pounds of sand. Make sure it's not filled all the way to the top; leave a quarter of the bag empty so that you can tie it up nice and tight. There's nothing worse than your bag breaking or opening up during a march.*

• *A daypack that fits snug against your back and does not have any slack in it. Fill it with the 30-pound sand bag.*

*Footwear: You can start out with tennis shoes or soft hiking boots, but I recommend progressing up to jungle boots.*

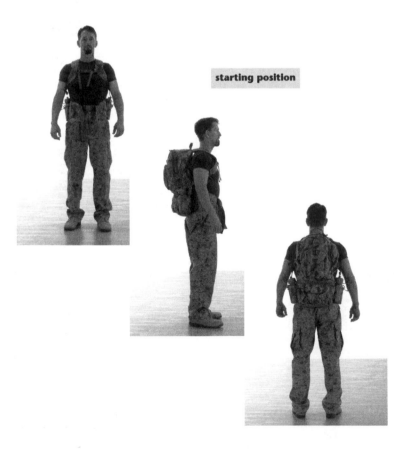

starting position

**STARTING POSITION:** Put on the daypack, making sure it fits well. You don't want the backpack bouncing up and down against your back and hips. To avoid any strain on your lower back, carry the bag high on your upper back, not slung low.

**1** Begin the Airborne Shuffle, which is a smooth march just under a slow jog. This keeps the impact low and reduces stress on the spine and knees. Basically, lift your feet just enough off the ground to move them without stubbing. Keep your arms relaxed with a 90-degree bend.

**TIP**
As you get stronger, you can progress from a 30-pound sand bag to 40 pounds to 60 pounds to 80 pounds.

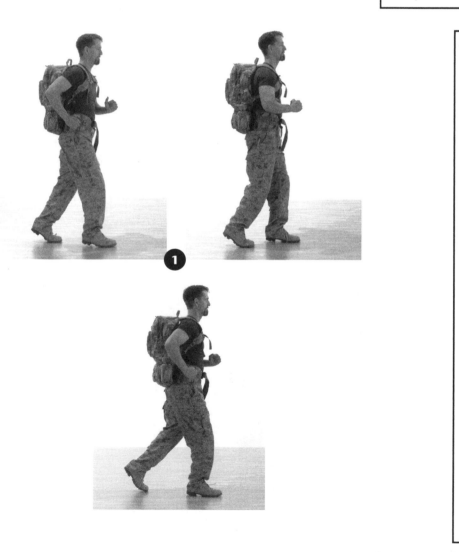

*Ill-fitting daypack:*

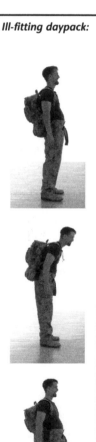

# hand to toes

*Special Ops Spin: No soldier will succeed during the obstacle course (especially the rope and wall climbs) if his abs are not strong. He won't have the strength to lift his legs to complete the obstacle.*

**STARTING POSITION:** Lie on your back and bring your feet to the ceiling so that your legs are 45 degrees to the floor; you can bend your knees slightly but not too much. Cross your ankles and rest your hands on your chest.

**starting position**

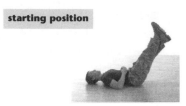

**1** Keeping your chin off your chest and driving with your shoulders, reach your hands toward your shoelaces, lifting your shoulder blades off the floor.

**2** Lower down to starting position, returning your hands to your chest.

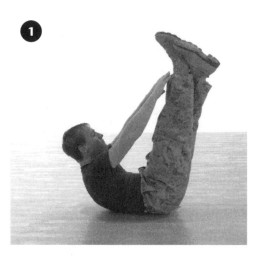

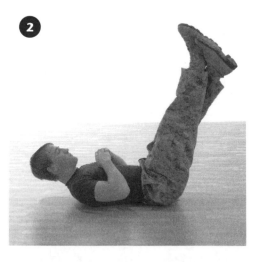

**TIP**

If you can't reach your shoelaces, aim at least for your lower shins.

# x sit-up

*Special Ops Spin: Core strength is essential and necessary to become an elite operator. For example, throwing a grenade is not all arm strength. Doing so requires a strong midsection so that you can coil and release for optimum distance and speed.*

*X Sit-Ups are a good all-round abdominal exercise but you have to reach the high reps to feel the burn. This is a four-count exercise such as 1-2-3-1, 1-2-3-2.*

**STARTING POSITION:** Lie on your back with your knees bent and feet on the ground. Touch your hands lightly to your ears.

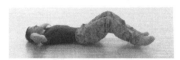

**starting position**

**1** Raise your shoulders four to six inches off the ground. Keep your shoulders off the ground during the entire movement.

**2** Raise your left leg so that it's 90 degrees from the ground, keeping your foot above your knee. Crunch into the final movement and try to touch your right elbow to your left knee. Do not bring your knee in towards your chest—do not compromise technique just because you cannot reach your elbow to your leg. Work on your strength so that you can eventually bring your elbow to your inner thigh.

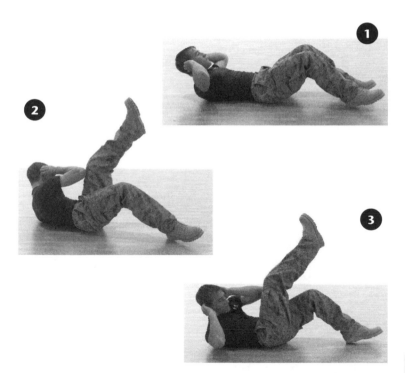

**3** Keeping your shoulders off the floor, lower your left leg to the floor and then raise your right. Touch your left elbow to your right knee. This is one rep.

**TIP**
You will rock your shoulders from side to side to complete your crunches but don't drop your shoulders back down at any time during the exercise.

# ranger crunch

*Special Ops Spin: Think about being loaded down with more gear than usual and fastroping into a hostile situation. You have a tight grip on the rope, your back is straight, and your legs are slightly elevated. Your strong abs and core make this possible.*

**STARTING POSITION:** Lie on the floor with your knees slightly bent and feet flat on the floor. Cross your arms and place your hands on your outer upper chest with your fingers barely touching your shoulders.

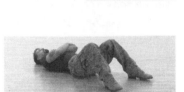

**starting position**

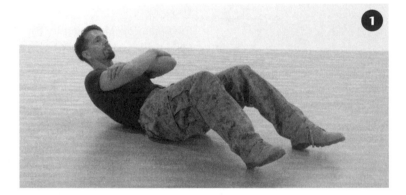

**1** Leading with your chin and shoulders, drive upward, lifting your shoulder blades just a few inches off the ground as you push your abs downward. Keep your chin away from your chest.

**2** Lower down to starting position.

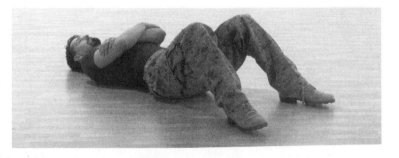

**TIP**
You don't have to lift your shoulders that high. The burn will be caused by how hard you crunch your ab muscles downward and towards your hips.

## supine bicycle

*Special Ops Spin: This movement is similar to a Special Ops operator sprinting up the stairs to the top of a building to provide cover fire for his fellow soldiers. You have to be quick and you must have quick core muscles.*

*This is a four-count exercise: 1-2-3-1, 1-2-3-2.*

**STARTING POSITION:** Lie on your back with your legs extended straight along the floor. Touch your hands lightly to your ears.

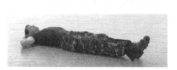

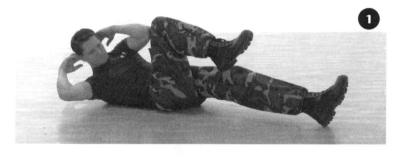

**1** Bend and lift your right leg 90 degrees towards your chest and raise your left elbow to meet it. Lift your shoulder blades slightly off the ground.

**2** Return your right foot to the ground before switching sides.

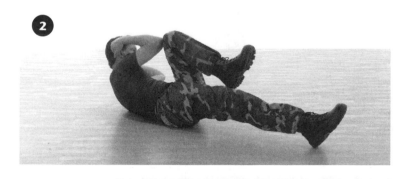

# hibberty jibberty

*Special Ops Spin: Think about being loaded down with more gear than usual and fastroping into a hostile situation. You have a tight grip on the rope, your back is straight, and your legs are slightly elevated. Your strong abs and core make this possible.*

**STARTING POSITION:** Lie on your back with your legs extended straight in front of you and six inches off the floor. Touch your hands lightly to your ears and lift your shoulder blades off the ground.

**starting position**

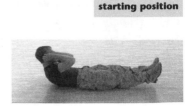

**1** As you bring your right leg in to a 90-degree position, simultaneously raise your upper body to meet it halfway. Touch your right knee to your right elbow.

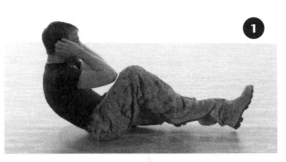

**2** Lower your upper and lower body back down to the starting position and then immediately move into the next rep, now using your left leg and elbow.

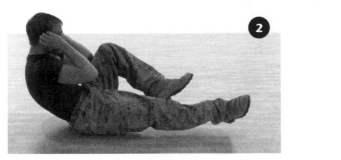

**3** In the final phase of this exercise, lower back down to starting position and then bring both your legs up together to the 90-degree position. Now touch your left elbow to your left knee and your right elbow to your right knee all at the same time. This will constitute one repetition.

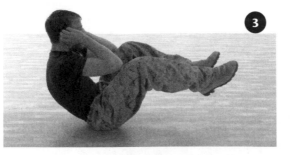

**TIP**
Do not jerk your body to get to the "up" position. This movement should be smooth and fluid.

## cross crunch

*Special Ops Spin: Core strength is essential and necessary to become an elite operator. For example, throwing a grenade is not all arm strength. Doing so requires a strong midsection so that you can coil and release for optimum distance and speed.*

**STARTING POSITION:** Lie on your back with your knees bent.

starting position

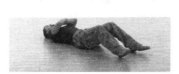

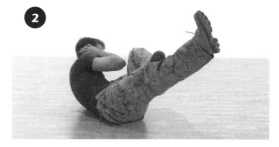

**1** Extend your right leg straight and raise it about two feet off the ground. Bend your left leg 90 degrees and place the foot on the inside of your right knee. Place your left hand on the ground for balance and your right hand lightly on your right ear. Keep your legs elevated throughout the exercise.

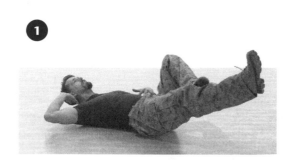

**2** Drive your right elbow into your left inner thigh so that you are crunching, not rotating, into position. Make sure not to bury your chin into your chest.

**3** Slowly lower your torso to the floor.

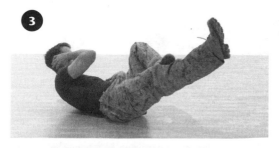

## obliques

*Special Ops Spin: Core strength is essential and necessary to become an elite operator. For example, throwing a grenade is not all arm strength. Doing so requires a strong midsection so that you can coil and release for optimum distance and speed.*

*Proper positioning of the hip is really important in terms of getting the most out of this exercise.*

**STARTING POSITION:** Lie on your right side with your legs and feet stacked on top of each other, slightly bent. Prop yourself up with your right elbow, keeping your right hand flat on the ground, and lightly touch your left ear with your left hand. Make sure the top part of your hip is rotated back far enough so that you're resting between your hip bone and your glute muscle. The top shoulder should be tilted slightly backward.

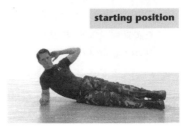

starting position

**1** Keeping your knees and feet together, raise them straight up about two feet and tuck your left elbow into your left thigh. Make sure not to come in towards your chest.

**2** Slowly lower down, lightly tapping the ground before moving into the next rep.

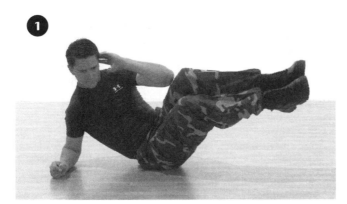

**1**

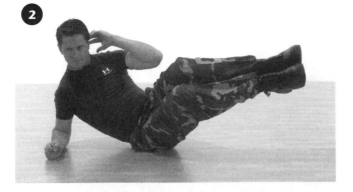

**2**

**TIPS**
• Don't lift your legs so high that you don't have to crunch to touch your elbow to your thigh.
• Don't bring your legs in towards your chest.
• If the exercise feels awkward, check your hip positioning.

*Special Ops Spin: Navy SEALs, Green Beret, Force Recon, and PJs are all scuba-qualified and need phenomenal leg strength to keep kicking. No one wants to throw off pace count, recovery time, or, worse, the mission.*

**STARTING POSITION:** Lie on your back and raise your hips off the ground. Place your hands underneath your tailbone, touching your fingers and thumbs together to form a diamond; allow a little space between your palms and the floor. Lower your tailbone onto your hands.

**starting position**

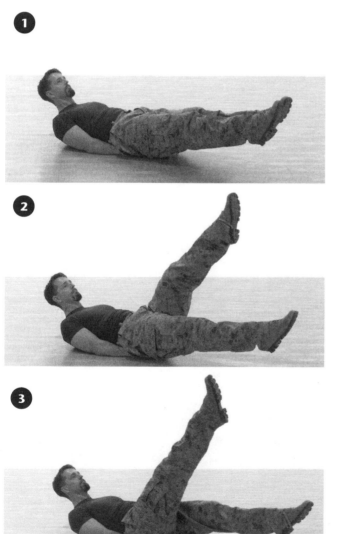

**1** Lift your head and shoulder blades off the ground, keeping your chin away from your chest by looking straight ahead.

**2** Straighten your legs and lift them 6 inches off the ground. Raise your left leg 36 inches, keeping your right leg off the ground. Press your abs downward and keep them tight to make this even more effective.

**3** Return to Step 1 and switch legs without letting your feet hit the ground. Continue keeping your legs straight and pressing your abs downward.

---

**TIP**
It is very important to keep your head and shoulders elevated during this exercise. If you're tired, lower your feet and head instead, rest, and then pick it up again.

## sky hop

*Special Ops Spin: Core strength is essential and necessary to become an elite operator. For example, throwing a grenade is not all arm strength. Doing so requires a strong midsection so that you can coil and release for optimum distance and speed.*

**STARTING POSITION:** Lie on your back with your knees bent and feet on the floor. Raise your hips and place your hands underneath your tailbone, touching your fingers and thumbs together to form a diamond; allow a little space between your palms and the floor. Now lower your tailbone onto your hands and extend your legs straight six inches off the floor. Lift your head and shoulder blades off the floor so that you can maintain a flat lower back during the entire movement.

**starting position**

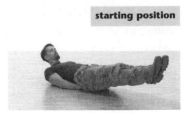

**1** Begin lifting your legs until they're perpendicular to the floor.

**2** Just as you're about to hit perpendicular, elevate your hips upward as high as you can.

**3** Slowly lower your legs to starting position, making sure that they do not drop too fast.

> **TIP**
> Use the same speed to raise your legs up and down.

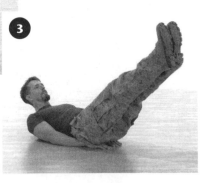

# lower ab crunch

*Special Ops Spin: Elite operators encounter numerous occasions when they need lower ab strength to lift their legs up and over a wall or object.*

**STARTING POSITION:** Sit with your legs straight and crossed at the ankles. Cross your arms and place your hands on your triceps, keeping your forearms parallel to the ground (*I Dream of Jeannie* style). Keep your abs tight throughout the movement to protect your lower back.

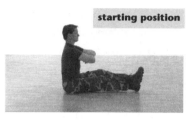

starting position

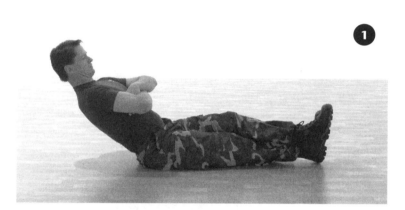

**1** Slowly lower yourself down about 45 degrees, remembering to keep your abs tight. Bring your arms down to your chest.

**2** Slowly raise yourself back up to starting position, lifting your arms away from your chest.

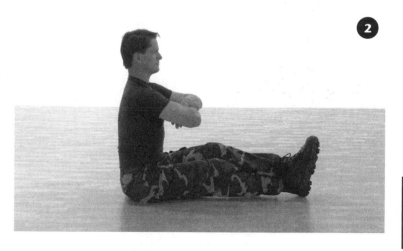

**TIP**
As you get stronger, you can lower all the way to the ground.

## scissor lift

*Special Ops Spin: Some branches call these Good Morning Darlings. They are extremely useful when it comes to swimming, sprinting, and long-distance running.*

**STARTING POSITION:** Lie on your back with your knees bent and feet on the floor. Raise your hips and place your hands underneath your tailbone, touching your fingers and thumbs together to form a diamond; allow a little space between your palms and the floor. Now lower your tailbone onto your hands and extend your legs along the floor.

**starting position**

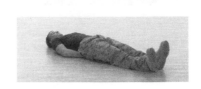

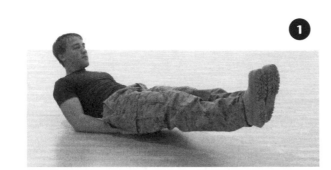

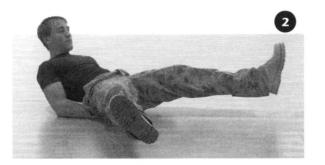

**1** Raise your legs six inches off the floor and lift your head and shoulder blades off the floor so that you can maintain a flat lower back during the entire movement. Keep your abs tight throughout the movement.

**2** Open your legs wider than shoulder width.

**3** Bring your feet back together, just lightly touching your feet together before you open them again.

# bench sit-up

*Special Ops Spin: Long marches, runs, and swims all rely on lower abs and hip flexors strength.*

*This is a very advanced exercise. If you have any back problems, I do not recommend it.*

**STARTING POSITION:** Sit on a bench so that your legs are extended along it and the upper part of your rear end is at the edge of the bench. Your partner holds onto or sits on your shins for stability. Cross your arms for balance and tighten your abs.

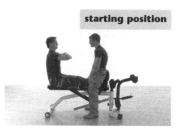
starting position

**1** Begin lowering your upper body, stopping when it lowers itself just past the level of the bench.

**2** Tighten your lower and upper abs to raise yourself back up past the 90-degree mark.

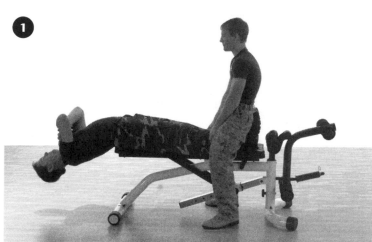
**1**

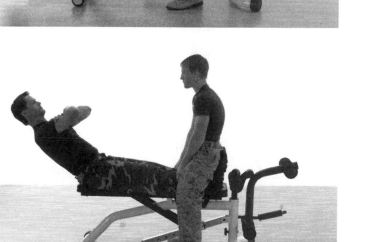
**2**

## fly my airplane

*Special Ops Spin: Fly My Airplane was used as a team-building exercise in the Army. Soldiers would take their helmets and place them under their stomachs. When the drill instructor yelled out "Fly your plane," they would lift every appendage and hold them straight out. If someone did not put out, the entire team would pay and continue suffering until that individual finally put out.*

*The main point of this exercise is endurance. It can be done on a helmet, medicine ball, or BOSU.*

**STARTING POSITION:** Lie face down with a helmet or medicine ball under your stomach. Stretch your arms out in front of you and your legs behind.

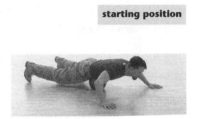

starting position

**1** Tighten every muscle in your body and then lift your arms and legs off the ground until they're sticking straight out from your hips and shoulders. Don't let them droop or rise too high.

**2** Slowly lower to starting position.

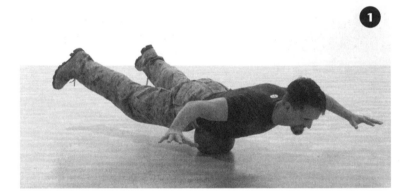

**1**

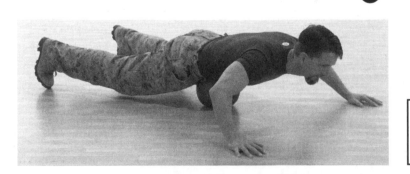

**2**

**TIP**
This can also be done with a pillow or balance ball.

# bench press

The Bench Press is a great old-school exercise that is excellent in developing chest size and strength. Just don't get caught up in maxing all the time. It's not about how much you bench but rather what the bench exercise develops. If it were all about the max then why does the NFL draft focus more on how many times a particular draftee can bench 225 pounds? Key points on the bench are the speed of reps, the intensity with which the bar comes off the chest, and proper positioning.

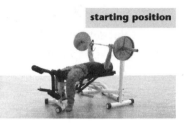

starting position

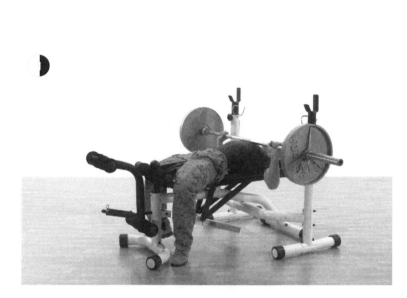

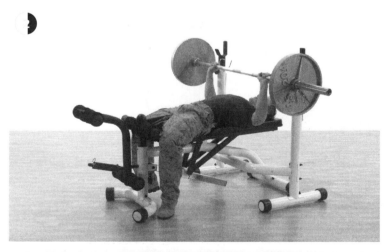

**STARTING POSITION:** Lie on the bench so that the bar is directly above your chest. With your hands slightly wider than your shoulders, wrap your hands and thumbs around the bar for increased hand strength and safety. It's best to be in a position that allows your arms to be 90 degrees once the bar reaches your chest. Keep your back on the bench and your feet on the floor throughout the exercise.

1 Safely lift the bar off the rack and slowly lower the bar to your chest. Do not come down too hard.

2 Once the bar hits your chest, drive it straight up. If the bar is above your mouth when you finish, readjust so that the bar is over your chest.

**TIPS**
• Do not lift your head; focus on your chest and triceps.
• Do not let your back raise off the bench.

# dumbbell fly

*I like to follow up the Bench Press with Dumbbell Flies, which really open up the chest. The emphasis here should be on slow methodical movement, not speed.*

**STARTING POSITION:** With a dumbbell in each hand, lie face up on a bench. Reach both hands to the ceiling, positioning your knuckles inward and keeping a slight bend in your elbows. To keep your arms in the right position throughout the entire movement, imagine that they are wrapping themselves around a barrel. Keep your back on the bench and your feet on the floor throughout the exercise.

**starting position**

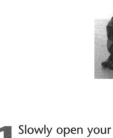

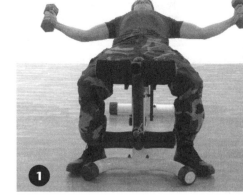

**1** Slowly open your arms out to the sides, making sure the dumbbells do not drop below your shoulders. Contract your chest muscles hard toward the end to help in the finishing of the movement and to help reverse your movement back to starting position.

**2** Maintaining the same speed, slowly return to starting position.

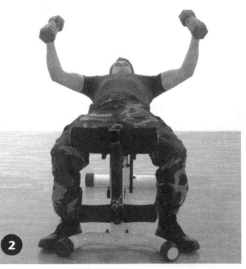

**TIPS**
• Do not bend your arms too much.
• Do not let your arms reach above your shoulders as you open up—keep them directly to the sides.

# triceps pull-down

*Along with dips, Triceps Pull-Down is one of the better exercises for developing your triceps. I like performing it with a solid bar one day and a rope the next to keep my body guessing.*

**STARTING POSITION:** Stand with your feet a little wider than shoulder width and hold the bar, keeping a 90-degree bend in your arms and your elbows tucked against your sides. Keep your hands out and away from your chest and stomach.

**starting position**

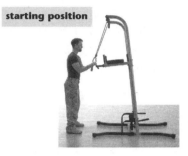

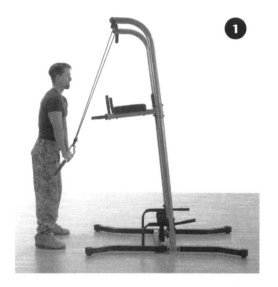

**1** Maintaining your elbow position, pull down until your arms are completely straight. The only body parts that move in this exercise are your hands and forearms. At the end of the pull-down, your wrists will flare out.

**2** On the way up, bring your wrists back together when you pass your belly button. Stop when your arms are at the 90-degree bend.

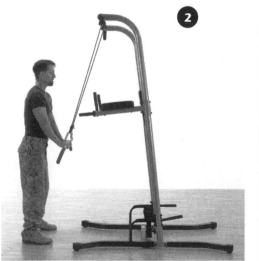

**TIP**
Do not rock or swing to start your next rep.

**MODIFICATION**
As the weight gets heavier, you might try putting one leg forward and the other leg back.

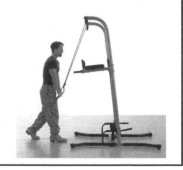

# skull crusher

*Proper hand, elbow, and ending position are the key to success with Skull Crushers. I like the inner grip better for this exercise, and a standard curl bar will keep your hands and wrists in the proper position throughout the movement.*

**STARTING POSITION:** Holding a curl bar in both hands, lie face up on a bench with your feet on the ground. Position your hands 6 to 8 inches apart on the bar and straighten your arms to the ceiling. Keep your elbows tucked in and your back flat on the bench throughout the exercise.

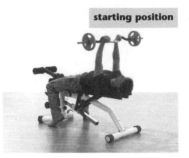
starting position

**1** Keeping your movement smooth and slow, bend your elbows and lower the bar until it's about an inch from your face, directly above your nose or eyebrows; do not bring the bar back over your head.

**2** Slowly return to starting position.

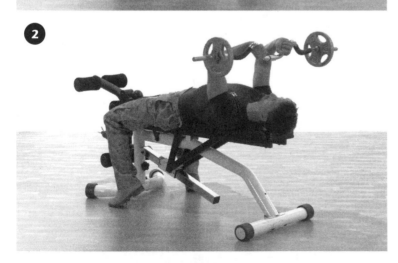

**1**

**2**

**TIPS**
• Always take the first rep the slowest to prepare your body for the stop and start.
• Do not let your elbows flare out.

# triceps kickback

*The key to Triceps Kickback is keeping your elbows in the up position while lowering your dumbbells to starting position. The only body part that should move during this exercise is your forearm. To further isolate the triceps, I like to place a twist at the end of the exercise.*

**STARTING POSITION:** With a dumbbell in your left hand, place your right knee on the edge of a flat bench while placing your right hand further down the bench. Bend your left arm until it's 90 degrees. Keep your elbow up and your shoulders squared throughout the exercise.

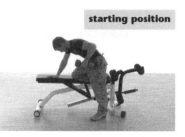
**starting position**

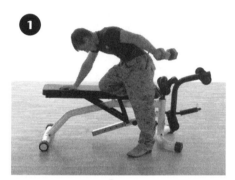

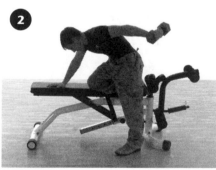

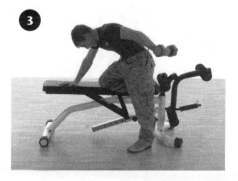

**1** Begin straightening your left arm. From the three-quarters position, rotate the top of the dumbbell inward until it forms a "T" with your arm.

**2** Straighten your arm completely.

**3** Without swinging your arm, return to starting position, making sure to keep your elbow up.

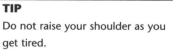
**TIP**
Do not raise your shoulder as you get tired.

# lat pull-down

If you can't perform pull-ups, this exercise will help develop the muscles you need to do so. It is also a great exercise to combine with your pull-ups.

**STARTING POSITION:** Sitting with your back to the machine, grab the bar about 2 to 4 inches from the end of the bar or, in some cases, where the bar bends. Wrap your thumbs around the bar. Look up and make sure that the point of the shoulders to where your hands rest on the bar form a V.

**starting position**

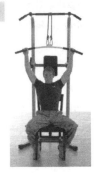

**1** Keeping good posture, drive the bar all the way down to the back of the head— rotate your shoulder blades inward while throwing your chest forward (this allows you to contract your back better).

**2** Maintaining the same speed, return to starting position; do not let the weight spring up on its own.

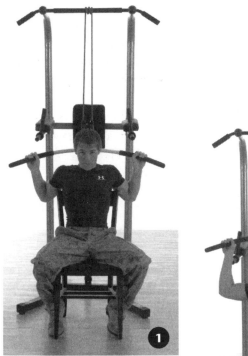

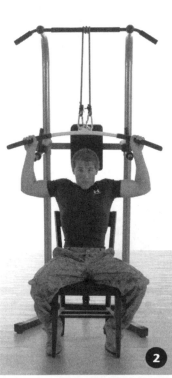

**TIP**
Always bring the bar down to the hairline for proper form.

# military press

*Military Press requires perfect technique for optimal results. I highly recommend a mirror nearby to see your technique.*

**STARTING POSITION:** Sit on a bench and hold a dumbbell in each hand, palms facing forward. The dumbbells should be above mouth height and touching. Make sure that your elbows are bent 90 degrees and that your elbows are slightly lower than your shoulders.

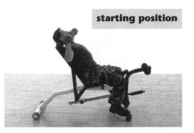

starting position

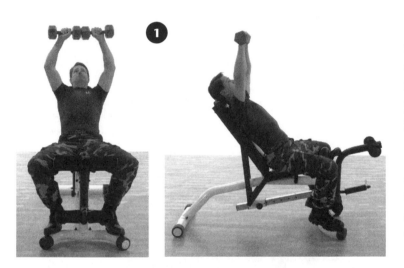

**1** Press up both dumbbells evenly, touching them together above your head; your elbows should have a slight bend at the top. Do not let your hands go too far behind your head.

**2** Maintaining the same speed, lower the dumbbells to starting position, making sure your hands don't open too wide or drop too low.

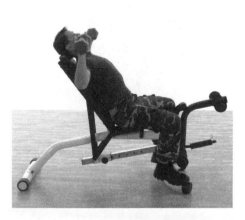

# shoulder rotation

*Shoulder Rotations work the full shoulder, front and back deltoids.*

**STARTING POSITION:** Stand with your feet wider than shoulder-width apart and your knees slightly bent. Your arms are along your sides, palms facing your body; hold a dumbbell in each hand. Tighten your abs to maintain a straight back throughout the exercise.

**starting position**

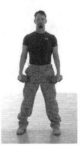

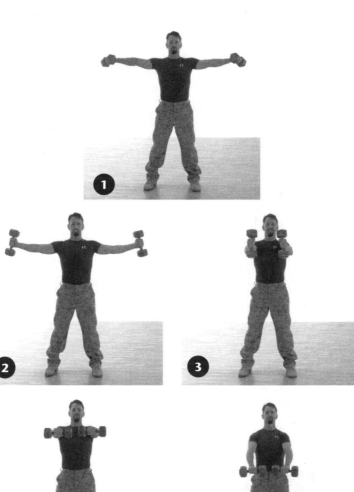

**1** Raise the dumbbells to shoulder height, keeping your arms as straight as possible.

**2-3** Once you reach shoulder height, rotate your palms forward and bring your hands together until they're a foot apart.

**4-5** When the dumbbells are directly in front of you, rotate your palms down and slowly lower the dumbbells to your sides, keeping your arms as straight as possible. Also make sure not to arch your back by tightening your abs more.

**TIP**
Fight the tendency to bend your arms, especially when you're tired.

# dumbbell shoulder raise

*This can be done with three positions—try them all to find out which one works best for your body. If you're lucky and every position feels good, you can hit every position during your repetitions. Go from side to V to front or alternate between sets, focusing on one position per set.*

**STARTING POSITION:** Stand with your feet wider than shoulder-width apart and your knees slightly bent. Your arms are along your sides, palms facing your body; hold a dumbbell in each hand. Tighten your abs to maintain a straight back throughout the exercise.

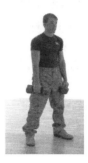

**1** Keeping your arms straight, raise the dumbbells out to the side until they're shoulder height.

**2** Maintaining the same speed, lower down to starting position.

**3** Keeping your arms straight, raise the dumbbells in front of you so that they're slightly wider than your shoulders; stop when they reach shoulder height.

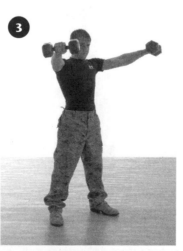

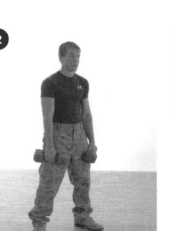

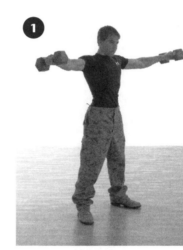

*(continued on page 126)*

## dumbbell shoulder raise (continued)

**4** Maintaining the same speed, lower down to starting position.

**5** Keeping your arms straight and your palms facing down, raise the dumbbells directly in front of you until they're shoulder height.

**6** Maintaining the same speed, lower down to starting position.

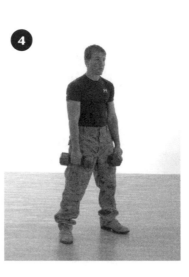

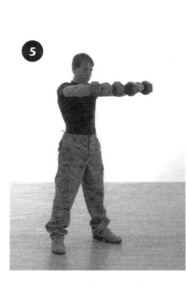

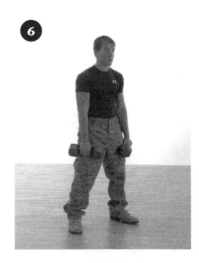

**VARIATION**
This can also be done by alternating arms instead of lifting both simultaneously.

# weighted lunge

The Weighted Lunge takes your lunges to another level. The only difference when it comes to weighted lunges is to watch the speed in which you come down into the lunge. There are three ways to do weighted lunges. My preferred method is to use a weighted vest; the best one I've found in terms of comfort and durability is by weightvest.com. Another tool is a curl bar (available at any sporting good store) with a towel wrapped around the middle. The third option is dumbbells, which are a fun way to add diversity to your lunges. With my wrestling team I would have them start out with 40-pound dumbbells in each hand.

**starting position**

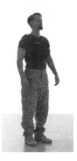

**STARTING POSITION:** Put on the weighted vest and stand with your feet about shoulder-width apart.

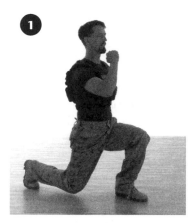

**1** Step forward with your left leg and bend your knee until it's 90 degrees—make sure your knee does not pass your toes; bring your right arm up to a 90-degree bend. Your right leg should be bent, with your knee one to two inches from the floor. Keep your shoulders back, your head up, and your back straight with each lunge.

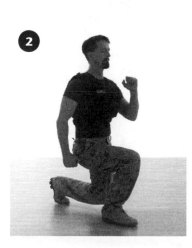

**2** Step forward with your right leg, bringing your left arm up.

**VARIATION 1**
Wrap a towel around the middle of the curl bar and place the bar behind your neck. Your hands should be a little wider than shoulder-width apart.

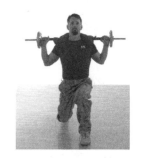

**VARIATION 2**
Holding a dumbbell in each hand, let them hang on either side.

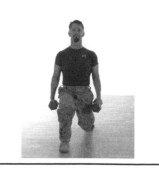

# preacher curl

*Preacher Curls can be done with an inner grip or a shoulder-width grip. Although it can be done with dumbbells, I recommend using a curl bar to get your wrists and hands in the right position. This can also be done on a machine with preacher pads.*

**STARTING POSITION:** Kneel behind a balance ball and place your elbows about shoulder-width apart on it. With your palms facing up, grip a curl bar with your hands shoulder-width apart.

**starting position**

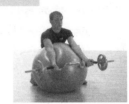

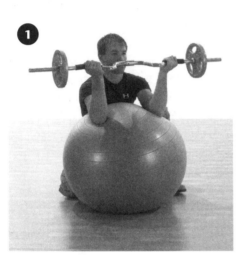

**1** Slowly curl the bar until it's three or four inches from your shoulders; make sure your elbows do not slide inward.

**2** Maintaining the same speed, lower down to starting position.

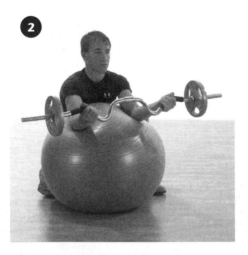

## VARIATION
If using a curl bar, you can also switch to the inner grips on the curl bar; if using dumbbells, press them together throughout the entire movement.

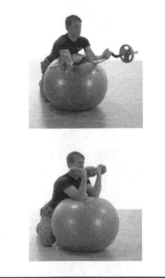

## seated dumbbell curl

*Forming a "T" at the top of your movement isolates your biceps and allows you to get much more out of this exercise.*

**STARTING POSITION:** Using an exercise bench that has an adjustable back, adjust the back of the bench just short of 90 degrees. Have a seat with your back flat against the bench and your abs tight. With your palms facing inward, let the dumbbells dead hang at your sides.

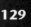

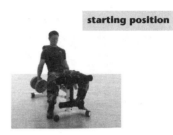
starting position

**1** Keeping your elbows by your sides, bring the right dumbbell up, leading with the thumb side of your hand.

**2** Once you are past your stomach, rotate your palm so that your palm faces your body and the dumbbell forms a "T" with your forearm. Continue curling the dumbbell, stopping a few inches before it touches your shoulder.

**3** Rotate your palm so that your thumb is up once again; lead with your pinky to return to starting position.

**4** Once your right arm is in starting position, raise the left dumbbell.

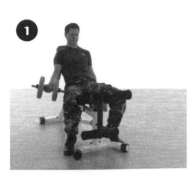

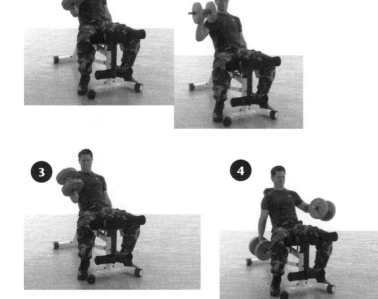

### VARIATION
To intensify the curl, you can rotate your palms downward before slowly lowering back to starting position.

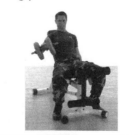

## curl bar—inner grip

*Curl Bar is a great way to finish off your biceps.*

*Putting a little throw forward in your shoulders at the very end helps keep your back straight. In other words, right before you get to the top, quickly and lightly thrust forward with the shoulders.*

**STARTING POSITION:** Stand with your feet wider than shoulder-width apart. Holding a curl bar with both hands, palms up, let your arms hang straight with a slight bend in your elbows. Tighten your abs to keep your back straight throughout the exercise.

**starting position**

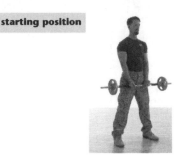

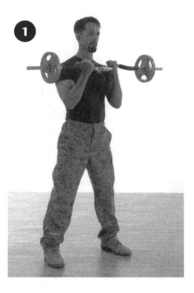

**1** Locking your elbows into your sides, lift the curl bar, stopping a few inches before it touches your shoulders.

**2** Slowly release down to starting position, making sure your arms are straight before continuing the next rep.

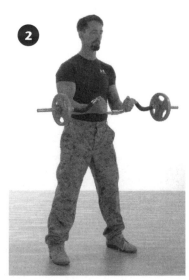

**TIP**
Do not arch your back—keep it straight by tightening your abs.

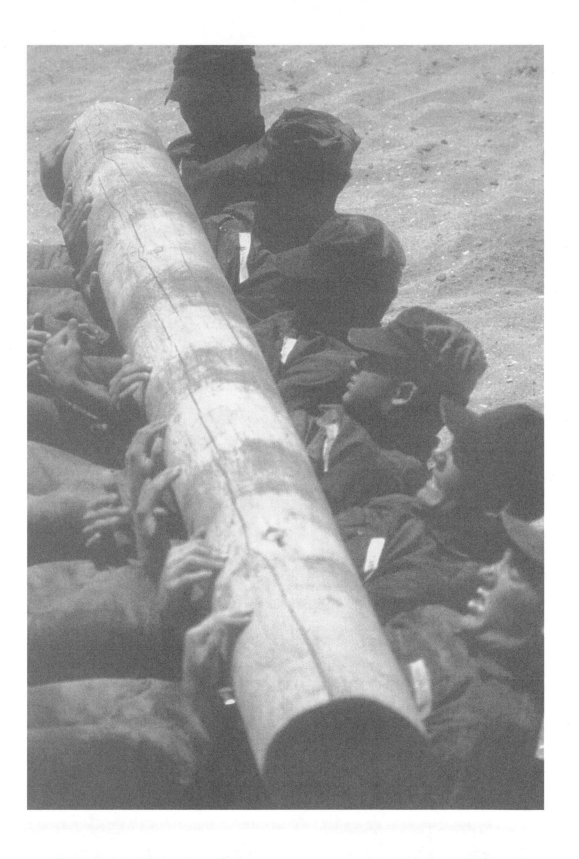

# index

# about the author

**MARK DE LISLE** has personally trained thousands of individuals with this workout. Originally from Folsom, California, he entered the U.S. Navy in 1990. In boot camp, he was given the opportunity to try out for the military's elite Navy SEAL training. Out of all the candidates who tried out, only two qualified. From a class of 130 SEAL trainees, after many grueling months, only 25 percent finished the training.

Upon graduation from Basic Underwater Demolition/SEAL School, Mark was assigned to SEAL Team 3, soon becoming Bravo Platoon's radio and communications expert and putting his training to the test in the Somalia conflict.

While in Somalia, Mark was constantly approached by sailors and Marines to put together a workout based on the SEAL training. The phenomenal results prompted Mark to go public, which led to national TV, magazine, newspaper and radio exposure that helped propel *Navy SEAL Workout* to become a bestseller.

Mark has also authored *Navy SEAL Exercises*, *Navy SEAL Breakthrough to Master Level Fitness*, and produced the DVD *Navy SEAL Workout*, System 1. He is now working on the *Navy SEAL Workout*, System 2 DVD.

# acknowledgments

Thanks to Andy Mogg for his exercise photos. It was a pleasure to work with him—he's a true professional and the best in his field.

A big thanks to Mark Divine and Tony Vernetti at www.navyseals.com for helping out with our interior shots. Navyseals.com is the best website for information about Navy SEALs, Special Operations information, products, and gear. Tell them Mark sent you and they will take good care of you.

Thanks to Mike De Lisle and Jeff Stephenson for their help on the photo shoot. They answered my call on a moment's notice and had my back. It was a lot of fun to finally do a project together with my little brother (sorry, Mike, you'll always be my little brother). Jeff, you're the best and I consider you a true friend. Congratulations on being two-time state wrestling champion.